Florence Lee
(650) 948-8722
17 Los Altos Ave.
Los Altos, CA. 94022

# *The* **New**
# **Sjogren's**
# **Syndrome**
# **Handbook**

EDITORS

## STEVEN CARSONS, MD
## ELAINE K. HARRIS

---

ASSOCIATE EDITORS

## Michael A. Lemp, MD
## Troy E. Daniels, DDS, MS

A Publication of the SJOGREN'S SYNDROME FOUNDATION

Medical Advisory Board Chairman STUART S. KASSAN, MD

Vice President for Research NORMAN TALAL, MD

# The New
# Sjogren's
# Syndrome
# Handbook

OXFORD UNIVERSITY PRESS

New York   Oxford   1998

Oxford University Press

Oxford    New York
Athens    Auckland    Bangkok    Bogotá    Buenos Aires
Calcutta    Cape Town    Chennai    Dar es Salaam    Delhi    Florence    Hong Kong
Istanbul    Karachi    Kuala Lumpur    Madrid    Melbourne
Mexico City    Mumbai    Nairobi    Paris    São Paulo
Singapore    Taipei    Tokyo    Toronto    Warsaw

and associated companies in
Berlin    Ibadan

Published by Oxford University Press, Inc.
198 Madison Avenue, New York, New York 10016

Oxford is a registered trademark of Oxford University Press

Library of Congress Cataloging-in-Publication Data

The new Sjogren's syndrome handbook / Steven Carsons, Elaine K. Harris, editors;
Michael A. Lemp and Troy E. Daniels, associate editors.
p. cm.
Includes bibliographical references and index.
ISBN 0-19-511724-7
1. Sjogren's syndrome—Popular works.   I. Carsons, Steven E.,
1950-   .   II. Harris, Elaine K.
RC647.5.S5S57   1998
616.97'8—DC21                                                    97-44421

3 5 7 9 8 6 4

Printed in the United States of America
on acid-free paper

*To all those people*
*who know they have Sjogren's syndrome*
*and to the countless others*
*who have yet to learn.*

# CONTENTS

# PREFACE

NEARLY TEN YEARS AGO, publication of *The Sjogren's Syndrome Handbook* began an era of dramatically increased awareness of Sjogren's syndrome by patients, their families, and physicians. Through the inspiration of Elaine Harris, founder of the Sjogren's Syndrome Foundation, *The Sjogren's Syndrome Handbook* was the first published work to bring together the cumulative knowledge and experience of the leading clinicians in the field to produce an in-depth yet practical reference that would be useful to patients, medical students, and practicing physicians in many disciplines. The impact on patient and public awareness, diagnosis, and improved treatment has been immeasurable. Some of the important milestones marking recognition of Sjogren's syndrome by public, governmental, and medical institutions are described in this volume in "A Personal Note on Sjogren's Syndrome."

In the time that has passed since publication of *The Sjogren's Syndrome Handbook*, there has been much accomplished in the development of new approaches to treatment and in our understanding of the biological causes of Sjogren's syndrome. Our readers have also given us many good suggestions concerning additional areas they would like covered in the *Handbook*. *The New Sjogren's Syndrome Handbook* is the product of these advances, accomplishments, and suggestions. Original chapters have been revised by their authors; new diagnostic and therapeutic developments have been added. The organization of the major sections of the *Handbook* has been modified to more closely reflect modern clinical approaches to Sjogren's syndrome and to accommodate the increased volume of information contained in this new edition. The overview section has been enhanced by the addition of a chapter entitled "Who Gets Sjogren's Syndrome?"—an exploration of the interplay between genetics and autoimmunity by Dr. Frank Arnett, a leading authority in the genetics of rheumatic diseases.

The section on extraglandular disorders now contains a chapter on lymphoma. Although a rare complication of Sjogren's syndrome, the relationship of lymphoma to Sjogren's is one of the most clinically important issues faced by the patient and the physician. The author, Norman Talal, in addition to being one of the clinical and research leaders in the field, has done the seminal work on the relationship of lymphoma to autoimmunity in Sjogren's syndrome. The prevalent problem of fibromyalgia, which commonly coexists with Sjogren's syndrome and other connective tissue disorders, is thoroughly reviewed by Dr. Rob Bennett, a rheumatologist with extensive clinical and research experience with fibromyalgia.

The section on gynecology and pregnancy is new as well, and it recognizes the extent of the impact of Sjogren's syndrome on all aspects of the life of a Sjogren's patient—who typically is female. The chapter on gynecology has been expanded and has a new coauthor, Dr. Lila Nachtigall. Dr. Jill Buyon has added information gleaned from her clinical studies on pregnancy and neonatal problems related to Sjogren's antibodies. A new chapter on the increasingly recognized antiphospholipid syndrome has been coauthored by Dr. Elise Belilos, a rheumatologist specializing in women's issues in connective tissue diseases.

The section on treatment and management contains four new contributions. Dr. Gary Rosenblum describes the approach to drug therapy for the systemic features of Sjogren's syndrome; his experience in geriatric rheumatology provides valuable experience in drug management especially for the middle-aged and older patient. Dr. Troy Daniels provides an invaluable guide to oral and dental care. Dr. Anne Lin describes the basic principles of medication use, and Dr. John Donlon provides important information on anesthetic management for all Sjogren's patients undergoing surgical procedures.

The editors and authors feel that *The New Sjogren's Syndrome Handbook* will provide our readers with the information necessary to intelligently recognize, diagnose, and treat Sjogren's syndrome as we move into the 21st century, an era which we are confident will see dramatic advances in finding an etiology and definitive treatment for Sjogren's syndrome and other autoimmune disorders.

*Steven Carsons, MD*
*January 1998*

# ACKNOWLEDGMENTS

THIS BOOK HAS BEEN nurtured and shaped over many months by many persons, all of whom share a great concern and compassion for those who have Sjogren's syndrome and those who care for these patients. At the heart of everyone's generosity are struggles, many questions, and an ongoing search for a solution for Sjogren's syndrome.

It was through founder Elaine Harris's tireless dedication and vision that the Sjogren's Syndrome Foundation was launched and grew to become the effective professional organization it is today. Mrs. Harris edited the first book on Sjogren's syndrome, *The Sjogren's Syndrome Handbook*, and began the work to develop this new edition of the *Handbook*. Thousands of readers and patients have benefited from her efforts. The new edition of the *Handbook* continued to take shape under the leadership of the former president of the Foundation, Jean Kahan.

During these times of change and growth for the Sjogren's Syndrome Foundation, Dr. Steven Carsons, as editor of the *Handbook*, has been steadfast in making this new edition possible. He was helped immeasurably by the associate editors, Dr. Michael Lemp in Ophthalmology and Dr. Troy Daniels in Dentistry and Oral Pathology. Most of all, the contributing authors have freely given their enthusiasm, their time, and their knowledge. For their gifts, the Sjogren's Syndrome Foundation is greatly indebted.

Steering the Foundation through this endeavor (and many others) are the Foundation's Medical Advisory Board Chairman, Dr. Stuart Kassan, and its Vice President for Research, Dr. Norman Talal. In addition, Dr. Philip Fox, Drs. Rolf and Tove Manthorpe, Dr. Dean Hart, and Diane

Chin provided invaluable advice during the creation and organization of the second edition.

The Foundation's Publications Committee, composed of Evelyn Bromet, Mary Anne Saathoff, and Michele Sinoway, played a vital role in bringing this book to fruition. In fact, all the members of the Board of Directors deserve high praise for their support. My special thanks go to Dr. Arthur Grayzel and Dr. Jeffrey W. Wilson for their advice, support, and encouragement in my work for the Foundation.

The staff of the Sjogren's Syndrome Foundation—Rita M. May (Executive Director), Alexis Stegemann, and Katherine Onderdonk—spent countless hours ensuring that this book would be the authoritative source for all those who want and need to know more about Sjogren's syndrome.

Finally, it is the membership of the Sjogren's Syndrome Foundation, who inspired this book and contributed a wealth of ideas and suggestions, that made Chapter 26 an indispensable guide to a better life for patients with Sjogren's syndrome.

The Board of Directors of the Sjogren's Syndrome Foundation thanks everyone who had and continues to have a hand in ensuring that Founder Elaine Harris's dream lives on, as expressed in the words of our Mission: "To educate patients and their families about Sjogren's syndrome, increase public and professional awareness of Sjogren's syndrome and encourage research in new treatments and a cure."

*Katherine Morland Hammitt*
*President, Sjogren's Syndrome Foundation*
*January 1998*

# A PERSONAL NOTE
# ON SJOGREN'S SYNDROME

A LITTLE OVER nine years ago, I wrote the Preface for the first edition of *The Sjogren's Syndrome Handbook*. That edition and this second edition represent milestones not only for Sjogren's syndrome patients and their families but also for the health professionals who treat these patients. Professionals have become aware that it is much easier to successfully treat a well-informed Sjogren's syndrome patient. Since 1982, when I was diagnosed with Sjogren's syndrome, when literally no informative patient literature existed, we have seen an ever-increasing number of patient-focused and professional-focused publications on Sjogren's syndrome and its many manifestations.

When first diagnosed, I was overwhelmed by feelings of both isolation and frustration. Can you imagine not knowing or not being able to contact another person with Sjogren's syndrome? Being unable to ask for the names of knowledgeable and empathetic physicians and dentists in your area? Having no source of basic information on current topics and resources such as the Sjogren Syndrome Foundation's *Moisture Seekers* newsletter? The absence of such resources prompted me to discuss this problem with three very supportive doctors who were taking care of me at the time. With the cooperation of these doctors and assistance from the New York chapter of the Arthritis Foundation, I was able to launch the first Sjogren's syndrome patient-support organization in the United States. It was initially called The Moisture Seekers. In 1985, we were incorporated and received status as a not-for-profit charitable organization. We changed the organization's name to the Sjogren's

Syndrome Foundation, but retained the name "The Moisture Seekers" for the now widely acclaimed newsletter.

For persons with Sjogren's syndrome, knowledge about managing the disease is the key to a more comfortable life. This knowledge has many aspects. Not only is it important for patients to be knowledgeable, but their friends, family, and the public also need to know what Sjogren's syndrome is. Most people today have never heard of this condition, although they are acquainted with some of its manifestations such as dry eye, dry mouth, and dry nose. They are surprised to learn that these manifestations, plus feelings of malaise, fatigue, and aching all over can be symptomatic of an autoimmune disorder for which there is currently no cure. Others, who may have heard of it, believe that it is primarily a disease of menopausal and post-menopausal women. Today we know that although the majority of Sjogren's syndrome patients are diagnosed after menopause, the condition may start years before, with symptoms developing slowly and insidiously. Furthermore, although Sjogren's syndrome occurs nine times more frequently in women, men do develop it, often in a fairly severe form—all the more reason for making the public aware of Sjogren's syndrome and its many manifestations.

We must educate people about Sjogren's syndrome. Amy Langer, the executive director of the National Alliance of Breast Cancer Organizations states, "We've learned that if you want your disease to be dealt with, you go and you talk about it and you market it and you visit and you stomp and you write letters and you do it." After the publication of the first edition of The Sjogren's Syndrome Handbook, a member who lives in Fairfax County, Virginia, was determined that every public library in her county should own a copy of the handbook; by going from library to library with the book and other Sjogren's syndrome literature, she fulfilled her resolution.

Never underestimate the power of the printed word. The Sjogren's Syndrome Foundation received its first big public awareness break in the spring of 1984 when an article on our organization appeared in the Long Island Section of a Sunday issue of the New York Times. That article was cut, copied, mailed, and faxed all over the United States, and resulted in the start shortly thereafter, of branches in Washington, D.C.; Delaware Valley, Pennsylvania; and Seattle, Washington. In January 1989, when the first edition of the Handbook was about to be published, the National Institutes of Health in Washington convened an interinstitute professional conference on "The Many Faces of Sjogren's Syndrome." In preparation for that conference, the Office of Health Information Clearinghouse printed special bibliographies for both patients and professionals and the *FDA Consumer* magazine had an in depth article on Sjogren's syndrome. Such conferences generate professional interest; media coverage generates public awareness.

We must "market" Sjogren's syndrome to raise the level of public and medical awareness and foster biomedical research. When an article that you can tie to Sjogren's syndrome appears in a newspaper or magazine, write to the editor and/or the author. Educate them about Sjogren's syndrome. Write to the health columnist. Ask questions related to Sjogren's syndrome.

This new edition of the handbook contains the most current authoritative information on Sjogren's syndrome. As you read it, you will note a fair amount of new, scientifically accepted information on Sjogren's syndrome. As reported in *The Moisture Seekers* newsletter and in scientific journals, new theories are developing as to what triggers Sjogren's syndrome, and new medications are constantly being developed. If you are a patient, I urge you to participate in those clinical testing trials for which you are eligible. Each of us responds to a particular medication in a different way. Indeed, I believe it is imperative that each of us, whenever possible, becomes an active participant in such trials. It is exciting to be one of the subjects who responds positively to a new medication being tested. And then, during the long process of trial and marketing, you will develop a better understanding and appreciation of the many steps, costs, and problems between the conception, development, and marketing of a new drug.

To the many persons who have contributed chapters for this new edition, I express my deep appreciation, for myself and for everyone connected to and treating patients with Sjogren's syndrome. We thank you for your past efforts and are counting on you to continue your efforts on our behalf.

*Elaine K. Harris*
*Founder Sjogren's Syndrome Foundation*
*January 1998*

# CONTRIBUTORS

FRANK C. ARNETT, MD, Professor of Internal Medicine, University of Texas Health Science Center, Houston, TX

ELISE BELILOS, MD, Instructor of Medicine, State University of New York at Stony Brook, Attending Rheumatologist, Winthrop-University Hospital, Mineola, NY

ROBERT M. BENNETT, MD, FRCP, Professor of Medicine, Chairman, Division of Arthritis and Rheumatic Diseases, Oregon Health Sciences University, Portland, OR

JILL P. BUYON, MD, Assistant Professor of Medicine, New York University Medical Center, New York, NY

STEVEN CARSONS, MD, Associate Professor of Medicine, State University of New York at Stony Brook, Chief, Division of Rheumatology, Allergy and Immunology, Winthrop-University Hospital, Mineola, NY

TROY E. DANIELS, DDS, MS, Professor of Oral Medicine, Director, Sjogren's Syndrome Clinic, University of California at San Francisco

JOHN V. DONLON JR., MD, Associate Clinical Professor, Harvard Medical School, Chief, Anesthesia Department, Massachusetts Eye and Ear Infirmary, Boston, MA

DAVID ESKREIS, MD, FACP, FACG, Clinical Instructor of Medicine, New York University, New York, NY

R. LINSY FARRIS, MD, Assistant Professor of Ophthalmology, College of Physicians and Surgeons, Columbia University, New York, NY

ROBERT I. FOX, MD, PH.D, Department of Rheumatology, Scripps Clinic and Research Foundation, La Jolla, CA

MITCHELL FRIEDLAENDER, MD, Director, Cornea and External Disease Services, Scripps Clinic and Research Foundation, La Jolla, CA

ELAINE K. HARRIS, MA, Founder of the Sjogren's Syndrome Foundation Inc., Great Neck, NY

ROBERT J. KASSAN, MD, Medical Director, Elderly Interest Fund, Medivan, Pompano Beach, FL, Rheumatology Consultant, Veterans Administration, Ft. Lauderdale, FL

STUART S. KASSAN, MD, Clinical Professor of Medicine, University of Colorado Health Sciences Center, Denver, CO

PAUL B. LANG, MD, Clinical Associate Professor of Medicine, Cornell University Medical College, New York, NY

JOAN LEVY, MA, CCC/SLP, Associate Director, Hearing and Speech Center, Long Island Jewish Medical Center, New Hyde Park, NY

DANIEL M. LIBBY, MD, Clinical Associate Professor of Medicine, Cornell University Medical College, New York, NY

ANNE Y. F. LIN, PHARM. D, Associate Clinical Professor, Wilkes University School of Pharmacy, Wilkes-Barre, PA

IRWIN D. MANDEL, DDS, Professor of Dentistry Emeritus, School of Dental and Oral Surgery, Columbia University, New York, NY

RITA M. MAY, M.ED, Executive Director 1995–1997, Sjogren's Syndrome Foundation Inc., Jericho, NY

HARRY MOUTSOPOULOS, MD, FACP, FRCP, Professor of Pathophysiology, Director, Department of Pathophysiology, National University of Athens School of Medicine, Athens, Greece

LILA NACHTIGALL, MD, Professor of Obstetrics and Gynecology, New York University Medical Center, New York, NY

ERNEST NEWBRUN, DMD, PH.D, Professor Emeritus, School of Dentistry, University of California, San Francisco, CA

ROBERT H. PHILLIPS, PH.D, Clinical Psychologist, Center for Coping, Hicksville, NY

THOMAS T. PROVOST, MD, Noxell Professor, Chairman, Department of Dermatology, Johns Hopkins University, Baltimore, MD

ROGER M. ROSE, MD, Associate Professor of Otolaryngology, New York University College of Medicine, New York, NY

GARY ROSENBLUM, DO, Instructor of Medicine, State University of New York at Stony Brook, Attending Rheumatologist, Winthrop-University Hospital, Mineola, NY

JAMES J. SCIUBBA, DMD, PH.D, Professor of Oral Biology and Pathology, School of Dental Medicine, Health Sciences Center, State University of New York at Stony Brook; Chairman, Department of Dental Medicine, Long Island Jewish Medical Center, New Hyde Park, NY

HARRY SPIERA, MD, Clinical Professor of Medicine, Chief, Division of Rheumatology, Mount Sinai Medical Center, New York, NY

E. WILLIAM ST. CLAIR, MD, Associate Professor of Medicine, Division of Rheumatology, Allergy and Clinical Immunology, Director, Sjogren's Syndrome Clinic, Duke University Medical Center, Durham, NC

ALEXIS STEGEMANN, Editor, *The Moisture Seekers Newsletter*, Sjogren's Syndrome Foundation Inc., Jericho, NY

NORMAN TALAL, MD, Professor of Medicine and Microbiology, retired

JOHN J. WILLEMS, MD, Associate Clinical Professor, University of California at San Diego, Director, Vulvar Disease Clinic, Division of Obstetrics/Gynecology, Scripps Clinic and Research Foundation, La Jolla, CA

# *The* New
## Sjogren's
## Syndrome
## Handbook

# Overview

# 1 What Is Sjogren's Syndrome? An Overview

AS THE 20TH CENTURY draws to a close, it is fitting to look back and see how much progress has been made in understanding Sjogren's syndrome and to consider the bright future before us.

About 40 years ago, Sjogren's syndrome was classified as a chronic autoimmune rheumatic disease characterized by the sicca complex (decreased tears and saliva) and resulting in keratoconjunctivitis sicca (KCS or dry eyes) and xerostomia (dry mouth). Extensive research focused on the immune response and its abnormalities in Sjogren's syndrome. The symptoms of Sjogren's syndrome were outlined and appear in Table 1.

Scientists think of the immune system as the body's way of defending itself against disease. Immune system cells, called lymphocytes and plasma cells, protect the body by killing foreign organisms such as viruses and bacteria. In Sjogren's syndrome and several other autoimmune diseases, however, the immune system mistakes the body's own cells for alien invaders. We call this process autoimmunity.

In patients with Sjogren's syndrome, lymphocytes selectively destroy and replace moisture-producing glandular tissue, especially the salivary (saliva-producing) and lacrimal (tear-producing) glands, destroying their ability to produce saliva and tears. Individuals with Sjogren's syndrome make certain autoantibodies, such as rheumatoid factor (RF) and antinuclear antibodies (ANA), which can be detected in their blood.

Any material the immune system recognizes as foreign is called an antigen. Antigens provoke the immune system to produce antibodies,

---

**TABLE 1   SIGNS AND SYMPTOMS OF SJOGREN'S SYNDROME**

---

*Oral/Salivary Signs/Symptoms*

Dry mouth
Cracker sign (see "Salivary Symptoms" in this chapter)
Burning oral mucous membranes
Parotid gland hardening or enlargement
Dental caries (tooth decay)
Inflamed oral mucosa
Dry, sticky oral mucosal surfaces
Reduced stimulated and unstimulated salivary flow rates
Inflamed salivary glands found in minor biopsy
Increased frequency of chronic yeast infections

*Ocular Signs/Symptoms*

Foreign body sensation
Inability to tear
Abnormal visual intolerance to light
Low values on the unanesthetized Schirmer test (see Chapter 5)
Decreased tear breakup time (see Chapter 5)
Twisted filaments of mucus on the surface of the cornea (the transparent "watch
    crystal" layer on the front of the eye)
Decreased tears
Characteristic rose bengal test (see Chapter 5)

*Systemic or Extraglandular Signs/Symptoms*

Rheumatoid arthritis or other connective tissue diseases
Fatigue
Fever
Infiltration of autoantibodies into the lungs
Kidney, muscle, nerve, and liver disorders
Abnormal globulins (a class of proteins) in the blood
Excess gamma globulin
Rheumatoid factor (RF), antinuclear antibodies (ANA), Ro/SS-A, La/SS-B autoantibodies
    (see Chapter 3)

---

blood proteins that help kill microorganisms. The measles virus, for example, stimulates the immune system to generate antibodies against measles. In autoimmune diseases, the immune system, mistakenly recognizing the body's own tissues as antigens, makes autoantibodies that attack these tissues and organs as if they were foreign. This attack is much like the rejection of transplanted tissue when an organ is surgically transferred from one person to another.

Autoimmune rheumatic diseases include rheumatoid arthritis, systemic lupus erythematosus, scleroderma, polymyositis, and dermatomyositis. These disorders are cousins of Sjogren's syndrome. They may overlap but nonetheless can be clearly defined, often have distinctive autoantibodies (like Ro/SS-A and La/SS-B in Sjogren's syndrome), and may require systemic medications like corticosteroids and/or immunosuppressive drugs, which affect the body as a whole.

Advances have been made in understanding autoimmune diseases. Some combination of genetic, hormonal, possibly viral, and neuroendocrine factors may be involved in causing Sjogren's syndrome. The genetic predisposition is weak and relates, in part, to genes that regulate the normal immune response. No virus has yet been found to cause Sjogren's syndrome, but scientists continue to research this possibility. We now know that the female predominance of this and other autoimmune diseases is due to the ability of sex-specific hormones to modulate immunity. Male hormones (androgens) are natural immune suppressers and female hormones (estrogens) are natural immune enhancers. The role of stress in these diseases is also being studied in a new field called psychoneuroimmunology.

No longer considered a medical rarity, Sjogren's syndrome is seen in 15 percent of the 2.1 million patients with rheumatoid arthritis in the United States. Moreover, for every person in whom Sjogren's syndrome is associated with rheumatoid arthritis, there is probably another in whom it is not. Many Sjogren's syndrome patients go undetected, since symptoms may be mild and easily overlooked.

Only 50 percent of the patients referred for Sjogren's syndrome actually have an autoimmune disease. Oral and ocular dryness frequently have other causes, such as amyloidosis or secondary to the ingestion of certain drugs.

### Diagnosing Sjogren's Syndrome

A diagnosis of Sjogren's syndrome is made when two of the following three cardinal features are present: (1) definite KCS; (2) positive lip biopsy, confirming the presence of immune cells or lymphocytes as the cause for the dry mouth; and (3) an associated extraglandular connective tissue disease (joints, skin, muscles) or disorder such as rheumatoid arthritis or systemic lupus erythematosus, commonly known as lupus.

A clinician often defines Sjogren's syndrome as primary or secondary.

---

**TABLE 2   DISTINGUISHING THE CHARACTERISTICS OF PRIMARY AND SECONDARY SJOGREN'S SYNDROME**

---

*Primary Sjogren's Syndrome*

Definite KCS and a positive lip biopsy, confirming the presence of immune cells as the cause of dry mouth, with no evidence of any other underlying rheumatic disease

HLA-B8-DR3 positivity (see Chapter 3)

ANA to Ro/SS-A or La/SS-B (see Chapter 3)

*Secondary Sjogren's Syndrome*

Definite KCS and/or a positive lip biopsy, plus evidence of accompanying rheumatoid arthritis or another connective tissue disease

Immunogenetic and serological (blood) findings of accompanying disease (e.g., HLA-DR4 positivity if the patient has rheumatoid arthritis)

---

A diagnosis of primary Sjogren's syndrome requires both measurable KCS and a positive lip biopsy for invasive lymphocytes; no other connective tissue disease or rheumatic arthritis is present. A diagnosis of secondary Sjogren's syndrome requires connective tissue disease plus either KCS or a positive lip biopsy. There are also immunogenetic (referring to genetic factors that control the immune response), autoantibody, and clinical differences between these two categories of Sjogren's syndrome (Table 2).

More than 90 percent of Sjogren's syndrome patients are women, whose mean age is 50 years. Sjogren's syndrome occurs in all races and in children. Patients most commonly consult a physician because of (1) the slowly progressive development of dry eyes and/or dry mouth in an individual who already has chronic rheumatoid arthritis or (2) the more rapid development of severe dryness of the mouth and nose, often accompanied by parotid gland swelling in an otherwise healthy person. The parotid salivary glands are located near the ears. These are the glands that swell when one suffers from the mumps.

## Ocular Symptoms

The most common ocular (eye) symptom is a sensation described as "gritty" or "sandy" or of a foreign body in the eye. Other symptoms include burning and accumulation of thick, ropy strands of mucus at the inner corners of the eyelids, particularly on awakening. Individuals with KCS also experience decreased tearing, redness, sensitivity to light, eye fatigue, itching, and a "filmy" sensation that interferes with vision. These patients complain of eye discomfort and difficulty in reading or watching television. Inability to cry is an uncommon complaint, and lacrimal gland enlargement does not occur very often.

### Salivary Symptoms

The distressing manifestations of dry mouth include difficulty in chewing, swallowing, and speaking; adherence of food to the buccal (cheek) surfaces; abnormalities of taste or smell; fissures (cracks) of the tongue, mucous membranes, and lips, particularly at the corners of the mouth; the need for frequent ingestion of liquids, especially at mealtimes; and rampant tooth decay. These patients are unable to swallow a dry cracker or toast without ingesting fluids, and they express displeasure at the suggestion. This symptom has been called the cracker sign. Individuals who are aware of having a dry mouth may carry bottles of water or other lubricants with them. They may awaken at night for sips of water. The dentist may notice that fillings are loosening or breaking down abnormally quickly.

Dryness may also involve the nose, throat, larynx (voice box), and tracheobronchial (windpipe and bronchial) tree and may lead to epistaxis (nosebleeds), hoarseness, recurrent otitis media (inflammation of the middle ear), bronchitis, or pneumonia. Half of the patients with Sjogren's syndrome have enlarged parotid glands, often recurrent and symmetrical and sometimes accompanied by fever, tenderness, or erythema (redness of the skin). Complicating infections are rare. Rapid fluctuations in gland size are expected, but a particularly hard or nodular gland may suggest a tumor, usually noncancerous.

### An Outline of Systemic or Extraglandular Symptoms

The arthritis of Sjogren's syndrome resembles classic rheumatoid arthritis in many of its features. Dry eyes can be expected to develop in 10–15 percent of patients with rheumatoid arthritis. Patients with sicca complex (dry eyes accompanying dry mouth) may experience joint pain and morning stiffness, without joint deformity. Fluctuations in the arthritis are not accompanied by similar fluctuations in the sicca symptoms.

Patients frequently experience skin dryness, vaginal dryness, and allergic drug eruptions. Red spots, called purpura, sometimes preceded by itching, may come and go on the patient's legs. Nephritis (kidney inflammation) rarely develops and suggests coexisting lupus. Severe muscle weakness may be an early symptom leading to a diagnosis of polymyositis (a simultaneous inflammation of many muscles). Muscle tenderness is an unusual finding. Involvement of peripheral nerves (nerves other than those found in the brain or spinal cord) may cause symptoms of neuropathy described by a patient as numbness or tingling.

For an in-depth discussion of systemic diseases, see Chapters 9–16.

### Immunogenic and Autoantibody Tests

Tissue typing tests, originally developed for organ transplantation, identify specific genetic sequences. These tests are similar to blood typing tests. Researchers have found that patients with rheumatoid arthritis factor and Sjogren's syndrome (secondary Sjogren's syndrome since rheumatoid arthritis is a connective tissue disease), like patients with rheumatoid arthritis alone, test positively for the HLA-DR4 gene, which determines a particular tissue type.

Interestingly, researchers have found that patients with primary Sjogren's syndrome test positively for a different gene: HLA-B8-DR3. People with lupus generally test positively for this gene.

Despite these genetic associations, simple genetic factors or patterns (hereditary) do not determine who will develop Sjogren's syndrome and who will not. Although it has been observed that groups of autoimmune diseases occur in families, the possibility of inheriting or passing on Sjogren's syndrome to one's children is not strong. If you have Sjogren's syndrome, it does not mean that your children necessarily will have the disease.

Blood tests that can specify a particular rheumatic disease and distinguish between autoimmune diseases await future research and development. Until then, tests developed to detect the autoantibodies common in several rheumatic diseases help distinguish between secondary and primary Sjogren's syndrome. These tests for particular ANAs have a different profile for each rheumatic disease, including Sjogren's syndrome, and help distinguish primary from secondary Sjogren's syndrome. Autoantibodies called SS-B (or La/SS) are found in the blood of the majority of patients with primary Sjogren's syndrome. They are also found in lupus patients, particularly when Sjogren's syndrome is also present. Autoantibodies known as SS-A (or Ro/SS) are also associated with primary Sjogren's syndrome but may occur in lupus as well.

## Recent Progress in Studying Sjogren's Syndrome

Biomedical science is moving quickly to narrow the gap between where we are and where we want to be in finding a cure for Sjogren's syndrome. Three major and interconnected areas of work are important for consideration:

1 *Lymphocytes* communicate with each other through a series of protein molecules called cytokines. For example, one such protein molecule, interleukin-2 (IL-2), binds strongly to the IL-2 receptor but not to any other. By binding to specific receptor molecules on the cell's surface, cytokines play a powerful role in immune responses.

Some cytokines augment the immune response, while others dampen it. In autoimmune diseases like Sjogren's syndrome, there is an excessive and inappropriate response due to the production of large amounts of augmenting proinflammatory cytokines that can be measured in the salivary and lacrimal glands. The goals of therapy are to reduce these cytokines and restore normal and proper immune regulation. Much of this is still in the future.

Once cytokines react with their specific receptors, molecular signals are transmitted into the cell nucleus where specific genes become activated and their specific gene products are expressed as proteins. These proteins may carry out important specialized functions for the cell (e.g., production of antibodies, hormones, or other cytokines). More generalized functions include life cycle events that all cells have in common. Among these is a phenomenon called programmed cell death or apoptosis (also called altruistic cell death), in which a cell suicide mechanism is activated.

2 *Apoptosis* (programmed cell death) is under active investigation in cancer and acquired immunodeficiency syndrome (AIDS), as well as in cardiac, neurological, and rheumatological diseases. On the surface of the cell is a protein called fas, which triggers apoptosis. Ab-

normalities found in the fas gene in an autoimmune mouse used to study Sjogren's syndrome began a flurry of research activity on the role of apoptosis in Sjogren's syndrome patients, and abnormalities of apoptosis. Epithelial secretory cells die an apoptotic death resulting in decreased saliva. Cytokines may be responsible for the fas-dependent death of the cells in the gland. On the other hand, the ability of lymphocytes to die by apoptosis is blocked by a regulatory gene called bcl-2.

3  *Oncogenes* (cancer-causing genes) and their normal counterparts, proto-oncogenes (non-cancer-causing genes), regulate cell growth, cell division, apoptosis, and various other general cell functions. In keeping with the oncogene concept, the term autogene is used for new genes involved in autoimmune diseases. Fas and bcl-2 have been designated the first two autogenes.

These three related areas of research—lymphocytes, apoptosis, and oncogenes—will, hopefully, lead to new methods of treating Sjogren's syndrome patients by restoring normal immune response mechanisms.

# 2 What Causes Sjogren's Syndrome?

THERE ARE MANY different causes of dryness of the eyes and mouth. The term Sjogren's syndrome refers to dry eyes and dry mouth as a result of an "attack" on the glands that make tears and saliva. In addition to dry eyes and dry mouth, Sjogren's syndrome patients may have dryness in other parts of the body, such as skin, sinuses, upper airways, and vaginal tissues. They may also have additional systemic (bodywide) manifestations including rash and fatigue, as well as joint, nerve, and muscle pain. Sjogren's syndrome is divided into primary and secondary forms. In secondary Sjogren's syndrome, the dryness is associated with other well-defined autoimmune disorders such as rheumatoid arthritis, systemic lupus erythematosus, scleroderma, and polymyositis.

Sjogren's syndrome was first described in 1892 by Johannes von Mikulicz, a Polish surgeon. However, because the term Mikulicz syndrome was subsequently used to describe so many other disease processes (such as tuberculosis and lymphoma of the glands), it became meaningless. Henrik Sjogren first reported the characteristic eye findings in his rheumatoid arthritis patients in 1932, but his research was not generally appreciated until it was rediscovered in 1953 by two American investigators, William Morgan and Benjamin Castleman. Since then, many studies have been published about the clinical and laboratory features of Sjogren's syndrome patients.

**TABLE 3   COMPARISON OF DIFFERENT CRITERIA FOR THE DIAGNOSIS OF SJOGREN'S SYNDROME**

| Criteria | Lip Biopsy (Focus Score) Required for Diagnosis | Autoantibody (Anti-SS-A) Percent of Patients | Criteria Exclude Hepatitis C |
|---|---|---|---|
| San Francisco | >2* | | Yes |
| San Diego | >2 | 84 | Yes |
| European (EEC) | 1† | 20 | No |

* A focus refers to a cluster of 50 or more lymphocytes in a salivary gland biopsy; the average number of foci in a 4-mm² area of a salivary gland biopsy specimen is termed the focus score.

† Lip biopsy is not required in the EEC criteria, but a focus score of only 1 is described as characteristic.

## Controversy About the Criteria for the Diagnosis of Sjogren's Syndrome

There has been a great deal of controversy in the scientific literature about the criteria for the diagnosis of Sjogren's syndrome, which has resulted in confusion in clinical practice and in research to discover the underlying causes. The methods for measuring tear flow and abnormalities of the surface of the eye (a condition called keratoconjunctivitis sicca) are not controversial. The problem involves the objective evaluation of a dry mouth. The gold standard test for Sjogren's syndrome has been the minor salivary gland biopsy. However, other systems of classification have tried to find a basis for diagnosis that does not require a biopsy. A comparison of three different sets of criteria is shown in Table 3. For example, the San Francisco criteria require the presence of an abnormal minor salivary gland biopsy. The San Diego criteria can be fulfilled by either an abnormal minor salivary gland biopsy or characteristic autoantibodies (such as antibodies to Sjogren's syndrome–associated A or B antigen). In comparison, the European (EEC) criteria can be fulfilled in the absence of a positive biopsy or characteristic autoantibodies. As a result, many more patients fulfill the EEC criteria than either the San Diego or San Francisco criteria. For example, only about 15 percent of patients fulfilling the EEC criteria would fulfill the San Diego criteria. Also, patients with dryness due to hepatitis C infection or other known causes of dryness (such as certain drugs or other diseases) would be excluded from the San Diego criteria but would be included in the EEC criteria. Thus, a patient may be diagnosed as having or not having Sjogren's syndrome, depending on the criteria used.

Unfortunately, patients sometimes get caught in this semantic debate between physicians about the precise diagnosis. It is important that all patients with significant dryness be offered symptomatic treatment for this problem. However, a clear diagnosis is required before any type of systemic therapy is undertaken. Also, the incorrect classification of a patient as having Sjogren's syndrome may delay the identification of other important infections that have an entirely different treatment.

## Control of Salivation and Tearing by the Central Nervous System

To understand Sjogren's syndrome, it is necessary to review the normal pathways that lead to saliva or tear formation. This is shown schematically in Figure 1. Sensory input from the eye or mouth is carried by nerves to the brain (shown by the dashed lines in the figure). These nerve signals go to a portion of the brain called the medulla, where specialized regions for tearing (i.e., the lacrimatory nucleus) or salivation (i.e., the salvatory nucleus) are located. This area of the brain regulates a series of functions called the autonomic nervous system. Activities such as the rate of breathing, maintenance of blood vessel tone (i.e., blood pressure), and intestinal motility are performed automatically. Thus, it is not surprising that medications that affect blood pressure or intestinal motility can also cause dryness.

Areas of cognitive function (such as the sense of taste or smell) are located in the cortex of the brain. These areas also send signals to the salvatory and lacrimatory nuclei. Also, emotions such as stress, anxiety, and depression that are processed in the brain may send neural signals to the lacrimatory and salivary control regions in the brain; a signal is then sent from the brain to the glands (indicated by the solid lines in Figure 1).

Thus, we can think of dryness as a result of two different processes. First, the gland may be destroyed by the immune system and not be able to respond to the neural signal. This is partly the case in patients with Sjogren's syndrome where an immune response is directed against the glands. The destruction of the gland can be seen in biopsies of the salivary or lacrimal glands. In this regard, patients with Sjogren's syndrome

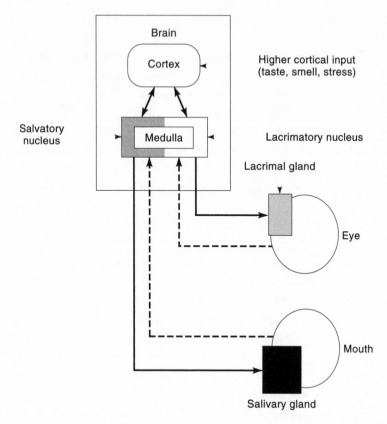

**Figure 1.** Schematic diagram for the neural control of tearing and salivation. The lacrimal and salivary glands are part of a larger functional unit that is connected by nerve fibers to the brain. Sensory stimuli from the eye or mouth surface and travel through nerves (called afferents) to the brain. This portion of the brain also receives input from higher brain centers (cortex) about taste and smell as well as depression and anxiety. The resulting "net" signal is sent back to the glands via a different set of nerves called "efferents." Any process that affects this basic "circuit" can lead to dryness of eyes and mouth.

share some similarities with patients with either thyroiditis (attack on the thyroid gland where thyroxin is produced) or "type I" diabetes (attack on the islet cells of the pancreas where insulin is made) as a result of immune attack. In this situation, attempts to prevent the immune system from mistakenly attacking the gland are the goal of present therapy and future research.

However, a second cause of decreased gland function in patients with dryness also may occur as a result of decreased nerve signals to the gland. If the signal from the brain to the gland is diminished, then the gland may be structurally intact but does not secrete in the absence of the correct neural stimulation. This type of dryness occurs in patients who have damage to the nerve to the glands of the eyes or mouth. Another cause of dryness is that certain areas of the brain do not give a correct signal to the nerves. This is the cause for the dryness associated with certain medications used to treat hypertension, seizures, or depression. When the drug is stopped, the gland function starts again and thus demonstrates that the gland has not been destroyed. Also, patients with depression or fibromyalgia syndrome may have dryness without significant infiltrates on their salivary gland biopsy. It is most likely that the neurochemical processes in the brain responsible for depression or fibromyalgia also influence the production of saliva and tears, leading to the symptoms that often mimic Sjogren's syndrome. However, the goal of treatment in this type of dryness is quite different from the attempts to control the immune system in Sjogren's syndrome. Since the problem is not due to overactivity of the immune system, attempts to depress the immune system are more likely to give side effects than benefit. Therefore, research is directed into stimulating the correct neural networks that lead to saliva production.

Although we have drawn a sharp distinction between neural causes of dryness and immune destruction of the salivary/lacrimal glands for the purpose of illustration, it is likely that there is a spectrum. For example, in Sjogren's syndrome patients, the salivary and lacrimal glands are partially destroyed by the immune system. However, the glands that still function may not work optimally because they are not receiving the proper signal from the central nervous system.

### Genes and Environment

Most researchers think that Sjogren's syndrome and other autoimmune diseases result from the interaction of specific genetic susceptibility genes with particular environmental agents, that is, things present in the person's surroundings. For example, a patient with the genetic susceptible gene HLA-DR3 may have an unusual immune response after infection with a particular virus or bacterium. As a result of these two factors, genes and environment, the immune system is tricked into mounting an immune attack on a particular target organ, such as the salivary glands.

Rheumatic fever is a well-known example of the immune system making this kind of identity mistake. During a streptococcal bacterial infection, usually a strep throat, the immune system mounts a strong attack against this bacterium. The immune system wipes out the bacterium, but 2 weeks later the patient may develop inflammation of the joints and heart. This happens because the immune system mistakenly identifies the normal cells lining the heart valve or joint lining as foreign (i.e., similar to a part of the bacteria), and it attacks and damages normal heart tissue.

No single gene causes Sjogren's syndrome. We know from studies of patients and their families, and from studies of animals with autoimmune disease, that at least four or five different genes are involved. Each of these genes might be considered an accelerating factor that comes into play when a susceptible individual encounters a relevant environmental agent such as a virus. It is likely that one or more of these risk genes are located on the female (i.e., X) chromosome, since there is a female predominance in Sjogren's syndrome. Because so many genes are involved, it has been difficult to determine precisely which genes are required. On the brighter side, this complicated requirement for multiple genes makes it unlikely that the patients' daughters, mother, or sisters will develop Sjogren's syndrome.

## A Viral Link?

What environmental agents initiate this process in Sjogren's syndrome? No one is sure. Indirect evidence suggests that viruses may play a role. Research interest has concentrated on the Epstein-Barr virus (EBV), a member of the herpesvirus family, which includes herpes simplex virus-1, the cause of cold sores, and varicella-zoster virus, the cause of chicken pox and shingles.

EBV infection is very common in the United States, affecting over 90 percent of the population by age 20. Initial EBV infection usually leads to a mild flu-like illness, occasionally with mildly swollen parotid glands. In most cases, the EBV infection is self-limited and clinical recovery is rapid. A minority of individuals develop more severe clinical symptoms of fatigue and swollen lymph glands, a condition known as infectious mononucleosis.

In almost everyone infected with EBV, including those with no symptoms, the virus establishes a "site of latency" or dormancy within the salivary gland, where it remains throughout life. Periodically, this latent

EBV may be reactivated, as indicated by the presence of EBV in the saliva of healthy individuals. This reactivation probably occurs more frequently in patients with immunological imbalances, such as during other viral infections that temporarily weaken the immune mechanisms that control EBV infections. When this viral reactivation occurs in patients with a particular pattern of susceptibility genes, a chronic inflammatory process such as Sjogren's syndrome may result. Although EBV has been suggested as one possible trigger in Sjogren's syndrome patients, the evidence for this hypothesis remains indirect and is not conclusive. At most, EBV serves as a trigger, since only a tiny amount of EBV is actually found in the Sjogren's syndrome gland. Further, it is important to reassure Sjogren's syndrome patients that since nearly all normal adult individuals harbor EBV, no one should worry about Sjogren's syndrome patients being carriers of this virus.

Some researchers believe that chronic fatigue syndrome is related to a so-called chronic EBV syndrome, but the existence of chronic EBV as a clinical entity and the relationship of chronic fatigue to the EBV virus remain highly controversial. Sjogren's syndrome is definitely not the same thing as chronic fatigue or chronic EBV syndromes.

## A Theory of How Sjogren's Syndrome Develops

As background, it is important to review the origin of the lymphocytes that constitute the body's immune system. Precursors of mature lymphocytes originate from stem cells in the bone marrow (Figure 2). Some of these precursors are destined to go to the thymus (an organ located in the chest) and thus are called T cells. The T cells mature in the thymus and undergo a process that removes any T cell that reacts with normal tissue proteins. Thus, the thymus teaches the T cell to distinguish between self and nonself. However, in patients with autoimmune disease, some T cells with self-reactivity escape the thymus and may enter the bloodstream to reach the tissues, where they contribute to an autoimmune disease. T cells are regulatory cells. In comparison, a different group of precursors in the bone marrow (called B cells) matures in the lymph nodes (Figure 2). These cells produce antibodies, proteins in the blood that react with foreign substances. The B cells are under regulation by T cells. In patients with autoimmune disorders, the B cells start to produce antibodies against normal tissue proteins. The protein that reacts with the antibody is also called an antigen. In Sjogren's syn-

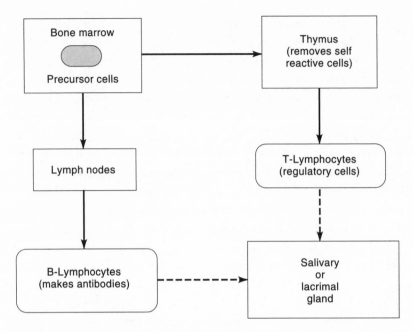

**Figure 2.** The origin of T lymphocytes and B lymphocytes in Sjogren's syndrome. In normals and in patients with autoimmune disorders, lymphocytes are derived from precursor cells (called stem cells) in the bone marrow. Some of these precursor cells leave the bone marrow and travel through the bloodstream to the thymus (an organ in the chest) where they undergo maturation. In the thymus, T cells with potential reactivity with self antigens are removed by a process of preprogrammed cell death called apoptosis. After thymic maturation, T lymphocytes enter the bloodstream and may eventually enter the salivary or lacrimal glands. If the T lymphocyte encounters a particular "self" antigen in the gland, the T lymphocyte becomes activated.

Precursor cells in the bone marrow may undergo maturation in the lymph nodes and other areas of the body to become antibody-producing cells called B lymphocytes. The B lymphocytes may produce IgG, IgA, or IgM antibodies. These antibodies may be directed against self antigens such as nuclear antigens (i.e., positive antinuclear antibody, ANA) or specific antigens associated with Sjogren's syndrome such as SS-A (Ro) or SS-B (La).

drome there are several different types of autoantibodies; the best characterized are antibodies against the nuclear antigens SS-A (Sjogren's syndrome–associated A antigen) or SS-B (Sjogren's syndrome–associated B antigen). These antigens are also called Ro and La. These are detected by blood tests and are the characteristic autoantibodies described in Table 3.

A characteristic feature of Sjogren's syndrome is the presence of lymphocytes in the minor salivary gland biopsy specimen. The microscopic appearance of a salivary gland biopsy specimen from a patient with

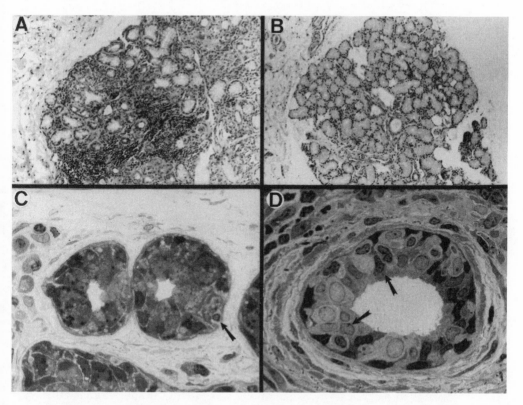

**Figure 3.** Microscopic appearance of minor salivary gland biopsy. Frame A shows a low-power view of a minor salivary gland biopsy from a patient with Sjogren's syndrome, while Frame B shows a normal minor salivary gland biopsy. Frame C shows lymphocytes (arrows) infiltrating a group of acinar cells (that create the water component of saliva), while Frame D shows lymphocytes infiltrating a duct (that carries the saliva from the gland to the mouth).

Sjogren's syndrome is shown in Figure 3A. The small, round cells that look like black circles are lymphocytes. The other cells that form rings are the glandular cells, including acinar cells that secrete saliva and ductal cells that carry the saliva to the mouth. In comparison, the normal salivary gland biopsy specimen shown in Figure 3B lacks these lymphocytic infiltrates. When the biopsy specimen in (A) is examined using higher magnification (C and D), the T cells (arrows) are shown to be immediately adjacent to the glandular (C) and ductal (D) cells. B cells also can be found in the salivary glands of Sjogren's syndrome patients but are fewer in number than the T cells.

One interesting feature of the biopsy specimen from a patient with

Sjogren's syndrome is that not all of the glandular cells have been destroyed (Figure 3A), as indicated by the rings of glandular cells surrounding the lymphoid infiltrate. Studies have shown that hormones released from the lymphocytes paralyze the nerves that send stimulatory signals to these residual glandular cells. Thus, the dryness in Sjogren's syndrome results from direct destruction of the gland cells plus paralysis of the remaining cells. The goal of therapy is to rescue these residual glandular cells and to get them to function at their optimal level.

The interaction of the T cell with the glandular cell is shown schematically in Figure 4. The T cell recognizes an antigen on the surface of the glandular cell. The interaction of the T cell with the glandular cell results from cell surface molecules expressed by each cell type. The T cell has a surface receptor called the T-cell antigen receptor (TCAR). The TCAR reacts with a cell surface molecule on the glandular cell called human leukocyte antigen DR (HLA-DR). There are many different types of HLA-DR (e.g., DR1, DR2, DR3, DR4), similar to the observation that the gene for a person's eye color may be black, blue, hazel, or other. The HLA-DR genes have evolved to allow either a high or a low response to particular infectious agents; they are called immune response genes. Only certain HLA-DR molecules (in particular HLA-DR3) predispose to Sjogren's syndrome among Caucasians, although other DR types are associated with Sjogren's syndrome in Japanese, Chinese, and black populations. Thus, HLA-DR is a genetic factor that predisposes to Sjogren's syndrome. The HLA-DR3 type in Caucasians is associated with a high response to SS-A and SS-B antigens.

The interaction of T cells and glandular cells, as shown in Figure 4, can result in the death of the glandular cell by a mechanism called apoptosis. In addition, the activated T cell and the glandular cell can release proinflammatory hormones (called cytokines) that cause local paralysis or death of the nerves that stimulate the remaining gland cells. Both of these processes result in the decreased saliva secretion and dryness that characterize patients with Sjogren's disease. The inflammatory cytokines may also escape from the gland and enter the bloodstream, where they stimulate other parts of the body to make proteins that result in an increased erythrocyte sedimentation rate (ESR) and C-reactive protein (CRP). These markers are tested by blood tests in Sjogren's syndrome patients to determine the disease activity. T cells in the gland also may act as helpers of B cells (Figure 4) and stimulate them to make antibod-

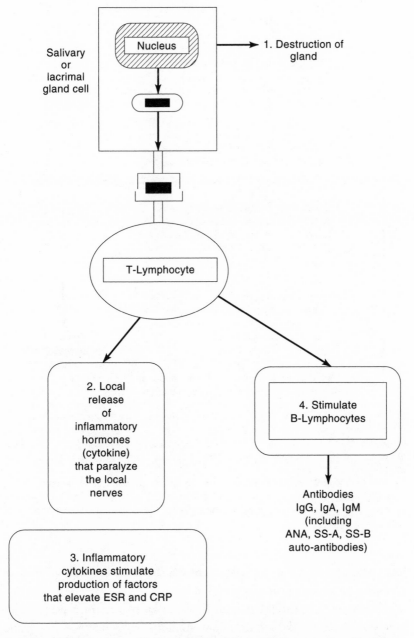

Salivary
or
lacrimal
gland cell

Nucleus

→ 1. Destruction of
gland

T-Lymphocyte

2. Local
release
of
inflammatory
hormones
(cytokine)
that paralyze
the local
nerves

4. Stimulate
B-Lymphocytes

Antibodies
IgG, IgA, IgM
(including
ANA, SS-A, SS-B
auto-antibodies)

3. Inflammatory
cytokines stimulate
production of factors
that elevate ESR and CRP

**Figure 4.** Overview of Sjogren's Syndrome. The initiation of disease begins with some extrinsic injury to the gland, which disrupts the glandular epithelial cells. As a result, lymphocytes infiltrate the gland and perpetuate the injury to both glandular cells and to the local nerve cells. The normal "feedback" mechanisms of the immune response are inadequate to terminate the response and the "inflammatory" cycle continues until salivary or lacrimal secretion is impaired.

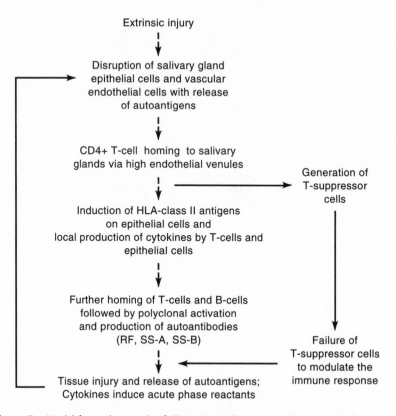

**Figure 5.** Model for pathogenesis of Sjögren's syndrome. An '' injury'' may disrupt the gland. This may be an exogenous factor (such as a virus or bacteria) or an endogenous factor (such as an inherited gene that causes the gland to function inadequately). The ''injured'' gland marks itself for recognition by the immune system by producing a protein called HLA (human lymphocyte antigen).

The HLA molecule holds self and foreign proteins in its groove in a manner that activates immune T cells. The result of interaction of T cells and the gland is the liberation of cytokines (lymphocyte and glandular hormones) and other factors that perpetuate the immune inflammatory response.

ies. Thus, blood tests that measure antibodies, ESR, and CRP give us an idea of what is happening in the glands.

Finally, new research has indicated that an important aspect of Sjogren's syndrome is the failure of autoimmune lymphocytes in the gland to die; again, this program of self-death is termed apoptosis. In other words, the immune system generates T cells, which are supposed to die by apoptosis after they have done their job. If the autoimmune T cells resist the normal process of apoptosis, they accumulate in large numbers in the glands and perpetuate the autoimmune response. Recent studies indicate that genetic factors may predispose to this resistance to apoptosis and provide another risk factor for developing Sjogren's syndrome. A goal of therapy is to develop drugs that will cause these autoimmune lymphocytes to undergo apoptosis while leaving the normal lymphocytes intact.

## Summary

Sjogren's syndrome results from a combination of genetic and environmental factors. There are at least four or five different genes, and they are only partly defined. HLA-DR, one of the genes that is important, is the same gene that is crucial in transplantation. Another important gene regulates the process of preprogrammed death of lymphocytes (i.e., apoptosis). The environmental cofactors in Sjogren's syndrome remain unclear. Indirect evidence favors a viral infection such as EBV. However, a variety of primary environmental causes may be sufficient to trigger the immune reaction, which then becomes a self-perpetuating process. An overview of the pathogenetic model is shown in Figure 5.

# 3 Who Gets Sjogren's Syndrome?

## Age, Sex, and Race

SJOGREN'S SYNDROME typically occurs in middle-aged women, yet it is not rare to see the disease in elderly or even young people, including children. Only 1 out of every 10 patients is a man. The reason for the striking female predilection is unknown, but estrogens are believed to play some role in promoting most of the autoimmune diseases. Certainly, one must question their importance in women who develop Sjogren's syndrome after menopause. Although information about racial differences in the occurrence of Sjogren's syndrome is incomplete, the disease can probably affect people of any race or ethnic background.

## Familial Occurrence

The cause of Sjogren's syndrome is not known, although several lines of evidence strongly suggest that genetic background plays some role. First, Sjogren's syndrome tends to cluster in families. Approximately 12 percent of patients have one or more relatives, usually female, with this disorder. Unlike purely genetic diseases, the pattern of inheritance in such families is not straightforward or predictable. Female relatives are nine times more likely to be affected than male relatives, and increasing age also appears to play a role. The risk for each first-degree female relative (parent, sibling, or child) appears to be approximately 1–3 percent. Actually, it is more likely that a relative will develop an autoimmune disease other than Sjogren's syndrome. Thyroid disorders are most common, usually hypothyroidism due to Hashimoto's thyroiditis or hyperthyroidism due to Graves' disease. Lupus also occurs more commonly in relatives of persons with Sjogren's syndrome. Less often, other autoimmune diseases such as rheumatoid arthritis, multiple sclerosis, or juvenile diabetes may develop in the families of persons with Sjogren's syndrome. Finally, blood tests are often positive in otherwise healthy relatives. Approximately 20 percent of relatives in a family with autoimmune disease, including Sjogren's syndrome, will have positive blood tests for antinuclear antibodies, rheumatoid factor, or anti-Ro (SS-A) and La (SS-B) but have no symptoms or other evidence of any autoimmune disease. Even over long periods of time (10–15 years), the majority of these relatives fail to develop any symptoms, although positive blood tests usually persist. Thus, family studies show a complex pattern of inheritance of autoimmunity (the immune system attacks the body's own cells) that strongly suggests that several different genes are necessary to produce disease. It is also likely that an environmental trigger, such as an infection, is required.

## HLA Genes

The second line of evidence for hereditary factors in Sjogren's syndrome is the discovery of some of the human genes that seem to play a role. They are termed major histocompatibility complex (MHC) or human leukocyte antigen (HLA) genes. There are many different HLA genes in the population. Therefore, in each individual, HLA genes are likely to be different from those of unrelated persons. Relatives may share some or none of the same HLA genes. The normal function of HLA is to direct the immune system's response to foreign challenges, such as bacterial or viral infections. Equally important, HLA genes keep the immune system from attacking normal, or self, components of the body. Therefore, persons receiving an organ transplant must be carefully matched to the donor's HLA types in order to fool the immune system into accepting the transplant as self. Otherwise, rejection by the immune system occurs. It is in this discrimination of self from non-self that the immune system fails in the autoimmune diseases.

Recently, the method by which HLA genes cause specific immune responses has been discovered. An HLA gene, such as DQ2, has a specific genetic code of DNA that is translated into a protein or molecule that does the actual work. This molecule is specifically shaped so that it can grasp certain proteins, either foreign (from bacteria, for example) or self (from

Ro, for example). The HLA molecule then presents this protein to T cells. If the protein is foreign, the T cells recognize it as such, and begin to attack it themselves and to cause antibodies to be made. If the protein is a self component, the T cells should remain quiet and ignore it. In autoimmune diseases, however, they treat normal self components as foreign and mount an immune attack. The reason remains a mystery.

In fact, in autoimmune disorders, certain HLA genes cause a very efficient and specific immune response to self components, such as the normal self proteins Ro and La, which typically occur in Sjogren's syndrome. This immune response to Ro and La results in the circulation of proteins in the blood (called antibodies), which are measured in the diagnostic testing of patients. The anti-Ro and La antibodies are also believed to directly cause some of the complications of Sjogren's syndrome. For example, pregnant women who carry anti-Ro and La may have babies who are born with a slow heartbeat (heart block) or a skin rash that is typical of lupus. These complications are due to the mother's anti-Ro and La antibodies, which have been transmitted to the infant via the placenta.

The HLA genes, which seem to influence Sjogren's syndrome and anti-Ro (SS-A) and La (SS-B) most strongly, are termed HLA-DQ alleles. It was once thought that the HLA-DR genes, specifically DR3 and DR2, were responsible. Now we know that the HLA-DQ2 and DQ6 alleles lie next to HLA-DR3 and DR2 in the genetic code and are the more likely culprits. Interestingly, while men with Sjogren's syndrome seem to have the same symptoms and complications as women, they usually do not have the HLA-DR and DQ genes (DQ2 and DQ6) or the typical antibodies of Sjogren's syndrome, namely, anti-Ro and La, ANA and RF. The HLA-DQ2 and DQ6 alleles are increased in patients with Sjogren's syndrome compared to normal individuals, especially in Western European whites and African Americans. The genetic association with HLA-DQ is strongest in persons who produce anti-Ro and La antibodies. Moreover, persons who inherit both HLA-DQ2 and DQ6 seem to have the highest blood levels of anti-Ro (SS-A) antibodies. This finding implies that a genetic contribution is made by both of the person's parents, HLA-DQ2 from one and DQ6 from the other. Thus, the inheritance pattern of Sjogren's syndrome is complex, even when we know some of the genes involved.

## Other Genes

The inheritance of HLA-DQ2 and DQ6 alone does not fully explain why people develop Sjogren's syndrome. When the HLA genes of patients' relatives are studied, it is not uncommon to find unaffected relatives who have exactly the same HLA-DQ genes as the patient. Thus, it seems very likely that additional genes must be inherited before the disease is expressed. Studies of other autoimmune diseases have shown this to be true. For example, in juvenile diabetes, which also requires certain HLA-DQ alleles, at least 11 different genes have been found that increase a person's susceptibility. The HLA genes contribute about 50 percent of this cumulative risk.

The third line of evidence supporting a genetic basis of Sjogren's syndrome comes from studies of animals with the disease. The most famous of these is the MRL-lpr mouse, which develops both Sjogren's syndrome and lupus. Recently, the major gene, called fas, and the role it plays in causing the disease in animals have been found. Basically, Fas is involved in a normal process called programmed cell death or apoptosis. The gene expresses itself in the thymus gland early in fetal development. This is the time when T cells are "educated" about what self is. Those T cells that react to self components are programmed by Fas to die; thus, by the time of birth, an infant should have only T cells that will react to foreign invaders. When the Fas gene does not perform its function, these self-reactive T cells survive and later cause autoimmune diseases. Studies are currently in progress to determine whether persons with Sjogren's syndrome have any genetic abnormalities in their Fas genes or in a variety of other genes involved in programmed cell death. When the defective Fas gene is replaced by a normal Fas gene in experimental mice, the animals no longer develop autoimmune disease. Such genetic manipulation of an animal model gives great hope for future uses of gene therapy in humans.

## Conclusions

Thus, to summarize, the person who is susceptible to Sjogren's syndrome is usually a woman. There is frequently a family history of one or more autoimmune diseases, most often thyroid disease or lupus. The patient usually has certain HLA genes, typically HLA-DQ2 and/or DQ6, and probably has inherited one or more other genes, the nature and functions of which are currently unknown. Finally, it is possible that the patient has been exposed to a common infection, which triggers auto-immunity against glandular tissue. This scenario may or may not be totally correct; however, given the rapid pace of medical discoveries, the true picture will probably be revealed soon.

# 4 The Medical Workup of Sjogren's Syndrome

INDIVIDUALS WITH Sjogren's syndrome have a variety of symptoms and complaints. Thus, they may initially consult more than one specialist. They may go to an ophthalmologist for their eye problems; an otolaryngologist (a physician specializing in ear, nose, and throat disorders) for their oral symptoms; and a dentist for problems with their teeth and salivary glands. These are the specialists who often diagnose Sjogren's syndrome.

Once Sjogren's syndrome is diagnosed, patients will probably be referred to an internist with a special interest in the disorder for a thorough evaluation. Rheumatologists and clinical immunologists are specialists with the most experience in treating Sjogren's syndrome patients.

### Medical Evaluation

The physician evaluating a patient for Sjogren's syndrome has four aims. The first is to assess the patient's general health status. The second is to determine whether the patient is one of the 50 percent of Sjogren's syndrome patients who has an associated connective tissue (joint, skin, muscle) disorder such as rheumatoid arthritis or systemic lupus erythematosus. The third is to search for other autoimmune organ system disorders that may be associated with Sjogren's syndrome, such as thyroid disease. The final purpose is to ascertain the patient's baseline immunological status.

The most important source of information for the physician is a comprehensive history, the patient's verbal account of the symptoms and signs that prompted the visit to the doctor.

Next, the physician may ask a series of questions that do not immediately appear to be directly related to Sjogren's syndrome. However, these questions are used to probe for subtle signs that may point to an associated connective tissue or immune disorder. Typically, the physician asks about joint aches, skin rashes, numbness of an extremity, or bruising and bleeding disorders.

The physician inquires about the health of family members, particularly those who may have autoimmune or connective tissue disorders.

The patient is also questioned about personal habits such as smoking, alcohol consumption, and use of medications, both those prescribed by other physicians and over-the-counter (OTC) or self-prescribed items. Although these questions may seem irrelevant, each detail is important. Common antihistamines in OTC allergy or cold remedies, for instance, may greatly increase dryness. The same is true of diuretics (water pills) and many other types of medication.

This discussion between physician and patient takes about 30 minutes, sometimes longer.

Next, the physician performs a general physical examination, including careful inspection of the eyes, mouth, and glands of the face and neck. The skin, joints, and scalp are examined, as well as the heart, lungs, abdomen, and extremities.

After completing the physical examination, the doctor orders routine blood tests to check the blood count, liver and kidney function, and blood sugar level. He or she tests the erythrocyte sedimentation rate (see the section on "Immunological Tests") and performs several immunological tests, described later in this chapter.

Because some patients with Sjogren's syndrome may have inflamed kidneys, urinalysis is important. The physician will also perform a chest x-ray to check the lungs for subtle signs of inflammation.

Following this comprehensive evaluation, the doctor either confers with other members of the team who have participated in the patient's care or reviews the records of other physicians.

After reviewing all available records, the doctor considers whether the patient has Sjogren's syndrome and whether any additional diagnostic tests are required to confirm the diagnosis.

### Additional Diagnostic Tests

If an ophthalmologist has not already performed the Schirmer test, (see Chapter 5), the physician will now do this simple screening examination. After placing a filter paper strip in the lower eyelid for a few minutes, he or she measures the degree of wetting with a ruler. This is concrete evidence that the eyes are dry.

As noted in other chapters, dry eyes and dry mouth, known as the sicca complex or dryness complex, do not constitute a diagnosis of Sjogren's syndrome. Dryness may be caused by many other factors, among which are allergies, climate, and medications.

Another eye test, usually performed by an ophthalmologist, is called the slit-lamp examination. This test tells the physician whether there is an accompanying inflammation in the external eye structures, such as the cornea.

When the eyes are dry and chronically inflamed, the doctor will diagnose keratoconjunctivitis sicca (KCS). KCS alone does not mean that the patient has Sjogren's syndrome. However, if the patient has KCS, swollen salivary glands, and/or a connective tissue disease, there is a high probability that Sjogren's syndrome is present.

The physician may evaluate salivary gland function. This is usually done simply by careful inspection of the mouth. In some instances, after stimulating saliva flow with a sour or acid substance, the doctor will collect and measure the saliva.

The salivary glands may be scanned with radioactive isotopes. After radioisotopes are injected into the bloodstream, scans of normal salivary glands show even uptake of the radioisotopes. Individuals with Sjogren's syndrome, however, have a patchy and diminished uptake. Results of the scans generally correlate with the degree of salivary flow.

For detailed evaluation of the salivary glands, the doctor may order x-ray procedures, but these are not often used in routine clinical practice.

In one x-ray test, called sialography, a dye is injected into the salivary duct opening the cheek so that the entire ductal pattern can be seen. In Sjogren's syndrome, chronic inflammation causes an abnormal pattern. Although this is a useful test when a stone blocking the duct is suspected of causing salivary symptoms, sialography is usually not necessary to diagnose Sjogren's syndrome. The procedure is uncomfortable and sometimes makes symptoms worse. It is usually not performed on Sjo-

TABLE 4   AUTOANTIBODIES PRESENT IN PATIENTS WITH
SJOGREN'S SYNDROME

| Antibody | Percent in SS | Other Disease Associations |
|----------|---------------|----------------------------|
| RF | 60–70 | RA, many others |
| ANA | 60–70 | SLE, others |
| SS-A | 70 | SLE (30 percent) |
| SS-B | 40 | SLE (15 percent) |
| Sm | Rare | SLE |
| RNP | Rare | MCTD* |

* MCTD, mixed connective tissue disease, an overlap syndrome.

gren's syndrome patients. Similar information may be obtained in a less invasive fashion by a sonogram or a magnetic resonance imaging study.

## Immunological Tests

Over the past several years, the discovery of many unique antibodies in the blood of Sjogren's syndrome patients has been helpful in diagnosing this condition.

During the evaluation, the physician usually performs several immunological tests. These tests are not diagnostic in themselves, but they are very helpful when evaluated in conjunction with the clinical examination.

Once immunological tests are performed during the initial evaluation, generally they are not repeated often. The following short list of currently used tests will help to demonstrate how the physician distinguishes Sjogren's syndrome from other immune disorders (Table 4).

- The erythrocyte sedimentation rate (ESR) is the simplest and most basic test routinely used to evaluate patients suspected of having an inflammatory or connective tissue disorder. The test measures how rapidly a column of blood settles. If the ESR is elevated, the person may have Sjogren's syndrome or an associated connective tissue disease. If the ESR is normal, a systemic inflammatory disorder (one involving many areas of the body) is less likely.

- Immunoglobulins or gamma globulins are normal blood proteins (antibodies) that protect the body from disease. In Sjogren's syndrome and connective tissue disorders, they are generally elevated. Some physicians repeat immunoglobulin tests to follow the activity of Sjogren's syndrome.

- The presence of antibodies called rheumatoid factor (RF) is important. Although RF is indicative of rheumatoid arthritis, it may also be found in individuals with other connective tissue diseases, as well as in those with Sjogren's syndrome. Therefore, a positive RF in a Sjogren's syndrome patient does not necessarily mean that the patient has rheumatoid arthritis.

- The antinuclear antibody (ANA) test is used to screen for systemic lupus erythematosus (SLE or lupus). Just as RF is not found exclusively in rheumatoid arthritis (RA) patients, ANA is not restricted to those with lupus. The ANA test may be positive in other connective tissue diseases, in Sjogren's syndrome, and even following the use of certain medications. Therefore, the sole finding of ANA in a Sjogren's syndrome patient does not mean that the individual also has lupus, especially if there are no other signs and symptoms of lupus.

- Recently, a group of antibodies called Sjogren's antibodies has been found relatively frequently in persons with Sjogren's syndrome. As discussed in other chapters, the two classes of Sjogren's antibodies, first discovered in the blood of persons with Sjogren's syndrome, are called SS-A or Ro and SS-B or La.

- SS-A/Ro antibodies occur in 60–70 percent of Sjogren's syndrome patients but are also found in those with other rheumatic or connective tissue disorders. SS-B/La antibodies are found in approximately 40 percent of persons with Sjogren's syndrome, more commonly in those who have primary Sjogren's syndrome, that is, with no accompanying connective tissue disease.

## Diagnostic Considerations

Before arriving at a diagnosis of Sjogren's syndrome, the physician will consider the possibility that the patient may have other disorders whose signs and symptoms mimic those of Sjogren's syndrome. Some of these disorders are discussed more fully in other chapters.

Allergies (see Chapter 15) may result in itching, redness, and a dry sensation in the eyes, nose, mouth, and throat that can mimic Sjogren's syndrome. Persons with human immunodeficiency virus (HIV) infection may develop lymphocyte accumulations in their salivary glands that can result in dryness and glandular swelling. These individuals are usually HIV-positive but SS-A/B-negative. Sarcoidosis is an immune-mediated inflammatory disorder of unknown cause that can cause accumulation of white blood cells in the tear and salivary glands resulting in glandular swelling and dryness. Sometimes an inflammatory eye disorder known as uveitis is caused by sarcoidosis. Sarcoidosis commonly involves the lungs, causing enlarged lymph nodes in the chest, and also causes arthritis. Amyloidosis is a disorder caused by deposition of an abnormal starchy protein (amyloid) throughout the body. If amyloid is deposited in the glands, it can result in their dysfunction, and dryness can occur. Finally, lymphoma (see Chapter 13) can involve the salivary glands and cause swelling and dryness in individuals who have never had or will ever develop Sjogren's syndrome.

## Relationship of Organ-Specific Autoimmunity to Sjogren's Syndrome

Sjogren's syndrome is often associated with other autoimmune disorders. As we know, when Sjogren's syndrome occurs with an autoimmune connective tissue disorder such as RA or SLE, we refer to it as secondary Sjogren's syndrome. Less well known, however, is the existence of another class of autoimmune disease that does not involve multiple organ systems (joint, skin, kidney, nerves) or the connective tissue disorders but rather a single organ (liver, lung, thyroid). This is termed organ-specific autoimmunity. The organ-specific autoimmune disorder most commonly associated with Sjogren's syndrome is autoimmune thyroiditis. In this condition, inflammatory cells may invade the thyroid gland; antibodies against thyroid tissue are produced as well. The antibodies can be detected in the blood and are useful as laboratory tests. Thyroiditis can result in either an overactive or an underactive thyroid gland. Symptoms of an overactive thyroid gland (hyperthyroidism) are sweating, palpitations, anxiety, diarrhea, and tremors. Symptoms of an underactive thyroid gland (hypothyroidism) include sluggishness, hoarse voice, dry skin, cold intolerance, and constipation. Physicians often check thyroid function tests and antithyroid antibodies in patients suspected of having Sjogren's syndrome. Other forms of organ-specific autoimmunity seen in association with Sjogren's syndrome are autoimmune liver disorders, especially primary biliary cirrhosis (see Chapter 11). Autoimmune hepatitis may also be seen. Autoimmune neurological diseases (multiple sclerosis and myasthenia gravis) also occur.

## How the Physician Diagnoses Sjogren's Syndrome

Once the physician has obtained all of the patient's test results, including the ophthalmological examination performed by the eye doctor and the oral exam performed by the ear, nose, and throat specialist and/ or the dentist, she or he is in a position to make a diagnosis of Sjogren's syndrome.

Before making a definite diagnosis, the doctor may recommend one last test, a small biopsy of the inner portion of the lip. This usually can be performed on an outpatient basis, often in a dentist's chair. The findings, reviewed by a pathologist, may give the physician an index of the inflammation and immunological activity in the salivary glands and indicate whether the patient has Sjogren's syndrome.

Patients and physicians should be aware that even among experts, there is no consensus on the exact criteria for Sjogren's syndrome. Currently, six investigative groups from diverse geographic areas (San Francisco, Tokyo, Copenhagen, La Jolla, Greece, and the European Community) have proposed sets of criteria that, if universally accepted, would become the diagnostic standard. Although generally similar, these criteria sets differ in their utilization of blood tests for autoantibodies (ANA, RF, SS-A/B) and in their absolute requirement for a minor salivary gland biopsy (necessary in three of six criteria sets). All criteria sets include KCS and some measure of salivary gland function. At this time, individual clinicians with experience in Sjogren's syndrome use some variation of these criteria to arrive at a diagnosis. In many circumstances, a biopsy is necessary to make a definitive diagnosis.

Once the diagnosis of Sjogren's syndrome has been made, it is extremely important that the ophthalmologist and dentist, as well as the internist, remain involved in the patient's care. The patient will see primarily the dentist or the physicians who specialize in the part of the body most affected by Sjogren's syndrome. Patients with chronic eye irritation and inflammation, for example, will see the ophthalmologist regularly. Those suffering from recurrent dental and oral problems will see the oral specialist.

If the patient does not feel well, the rheumatologist or immunologist will wish to do a reevaluation, perhaps performing a few blood tests to determine whether the new problem is related to Sjogren's syndrome and whether additional treatment is required.

Like everyone else, Sjogren's syndrome patients may have minor illnesses, such as colds, urinary tract infections, sprains, and muscle strains. New symptoms may not necessarily be associated with Sjogren's syndrome and may require only routine medical treatment.

Although Sjogren's syndrome is a chronic illness, nearly all patients can lead productive lives. Currently, most physicians specializing in Sjogren's syndrome prefer to treat their patients conservatively, using preparations to restore or stimulate moisture production locally. Because of chronic and potentially serious side effects, potent immunomodulating drugs, such as cortisone, are not routinely used to treat dryness or local swelling. These drugs are reserved for severe inflammation of vital organs.

Monitoring and treatment by an appropriate health care team will help the Sjogren's syndrome patient feel more comfortable and prevent avoidable complications.

# Major Gland
## Involvement

**R. Linsy Farris, MD**

**Mitchell Friedlaender, MD**

# 5  The Dry Eye

BLURRED VISION, intolerance of bright light, grittiness, burning, itching, and foreign body sensation are common symptoms of a dry eye.

Paradoxically, a feeling of excessive tearing may be associated with dry eye. If resting state tearing (the amount of tears present when the eyes are not being stimulated very much) is not enough to moisten the eye properly, the eye produces reflex tears. When resting state tears are increased, reflex tearing subsides. Reflex tears normally occur whenever the eye is irritated by a foreign body, a gust of wind, a blast of air from an air conditioner, or anything that dries the surface of the eye.

Dry eye patients often notice that their symptoms worsen as the day progresses. Malfunctioning lacrimal (tear) glands cannot keep up with normal evaporative losses. Evaporation exceeds the rate of tear production, and the integrity of the tear film deteriorates throughout the day.

Because the tear film is essential to providing a smooth surface on the front of the eye where light rays are focused, blurred vision is often one of the first signs of a dry eye. A dry, somewhat roughened surface scatters rays of light as they strike the eye, resulting in blurred vision. This is somewhat like looking through a dirty windshield.

Blinking several times to increase the tears on the surface of the cornea (the transparent structure up front, the "watch crystal" of the eye) will improve vision. So will any measure that increases the amount of moisture on the front of the cornea.

Providing increased moisture by means of artificial tear solutions may bring relief but will not cure a dry eye condition. Relief is temporary because artificial tears hydrate the tear film but evaporate or drain away easily unless the natural tear film is restored.

### Medical Care Is Important

Persons with dry eye symptoms should have a complete examination by an ophthalmologist, a physician specializing in eye disorders. The ophthalmologist will assess the condition and determine whether there is any ulceration, infection, or another ocular problem that, if left untreated, could endanger the patient's vision.

Patients frequently must search to find an ophthalmologist who has an interest in the dry eye and the patience to provide continuing care for a condition with no current cure.

Dry eye patients should be under the regular care of an ophthalmologist. They should have checkups at least every 6 months and possibly more frequently, depending on the severity of the symptoms and the state of the eye disease.

### What Are the Components of the Normal Tear Film?

Because the dry eye involves much more than inadequate tears, the diagnosis is not easy. An inadequate tear film may be caused by abnormalities in the composition of any of the three layers of the film itself, in the eyelids, or in the cornea.

The tear film is a three-layer structure made up of mucus and fatty substances, as well as water and proteins (essential chemical compounds of all cells). The higher concentration of mucus on the surface of the cornea is called the mucin layer. The middle, watery layer that makes up most of the tear film is the aqueous layer. The outer thin layer of fatty substances derived from the eyelids is the lipid layer.

The tear film is as complex as blood and other body secretions. Any one of its components may be affected by eye disorders or disease, disrupting the continuous, intact film of liquid on the surface of the cornea.

### What Is the Role of the Mucin Layer?

Mucin glands are scattered throughout the conjunctiva (the mucous membrane covering the outside of the eyeball and the lining of the lids). By continuously secreting mucin, these glands provide the mucin component of the tear film. Without adequate mucin lubrication, dry spots quickly develop on the cornea, leading to localized areas of tear deficiency. This stimulates corneal nerve endings, provoking the symptoms of dry eye described earlier.

## What Is the Role of the Aqueous Layer?

The main and accessory lacrimal glands deliver watery secretions into an accessory tear duct that empties into the upper conjunctiva, beneath the outer portion of the eyelid, and into the nasolacrimal tear duct. These watery secretions contain a variety of proteins, including lysozyme and lactoferrin, two of the antibacterial substances in tears that protect the eye against infections.

## What Is the Role of the Lipid Layer?

The fatty secretions of the tear film rest in a thin layer on the outer surface of the eye, protecting the eye by retarding evaporation of the tears. These fatty secretions work somewhat like paraffin placed on a jar of jelly. Lipid deficiency leads to excessive evaporation, which, in turn, leads to decreased tear volume and a dry eye.

In some cases, the fatty substances or lipids may be excessive, contaminating the underlying aqueous and mucin layers and resulting in dry spot formation. Normally, these three layers of the tear film appear to maintain a balance, preventing evaporation and continuously lubricating the surface of the cornea with tears.

## What Are the Roles of the Eyelids and the Corneal Surface?

In addition to the components in the three tear film layers, the distribution of tears by the eyelids is extremely important. This permits tears to moisten and smooth out the eye surface. The surface of the cornea must also be normal and intact to serve as a good foundation or base for the tear film.

Changes in the normal motion of the eyelids, as a result of an activity such as staring, cause excessive drying of the corneal surface. Neurological conditions that prevent spontaneous blinking are likely to produce a dry eye due to excessive evaporation. The corneal surface may also suffer from degenerations or diseases, called dystrophies, which may produce areas that cannot be resurfaced and covered by the normal tear film.

## Diagnostic Tests

The manifestations of dry eye are subtle and may not be evident to the physician when the eyes are examined. Several diagnostic tests help determine whether one has a dry eye condition.

Diagnostic tests of tear film abnormalities vary greatly in sensitivity (ability to obtain true-positive results in patients with a disease) and specificity (ability to determine normal persons free of disease). Very seldom do tests have both high sensitivity and high specificity.

When a set of criteria is used to compare a group of normal persons and a group of dry eye patients, all diagnostic tests will have an overlap of values, that is, a gray zone. This may obscure the true value and accuracy of the test. As a result, diagnostic tests are used only as a guide. The diagnosis is made by considering the person's history, symptoms, and physical examination for signs of dry eye, as well as by diagnostic tests.

In the final analysis, the diagnosis of dry eye is a judgment that becomes more definite as the physician's experience with the patient continues, both before and after various therapies are instituted.

### Slit-Lamp Examination

In testing for dry eye, it is particularly important to avoid any stimulation that would produce reflex tearing, thereby masking the condition. In the slit-lamp examination, which provides magnification without direct illumination, the eye can be viewed in its resting state and the basal tear volume examined.

A wedge of tears, called the inferior marginal tear strip, usually rests on the lower eyelid margin. Its size may be a guide to the total volume of tears. Excessive debris in the tear film may be apparent, as well as a more viscous-appearing tear film and low-grade inflammation of the conjunctiva.

### Schirmer Test

Perhaps one of the best-known tests for tear function, the Schirmer test, is easily performed, with or without a drop of anesthetic in the eye prior to the test. The only requirements are small strips of filter paper. When performed without anesthesia, this test may be viewed as a stress

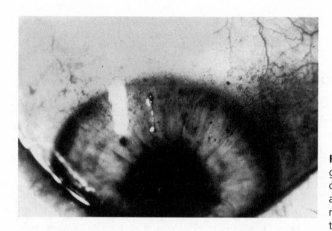

**Figure 6.** Rose bengal stains dry spots on the ocular surface and also mucous filaments that cling to the eye.

test because of the stimulation caused by the dry filter paper when it touches the eyelid and conjunctiva.

The amount of stimulation varies greatly in individual patients, resulting in immediate, complete wetting in some and only 4 mm or less of wetting in others. In addition to sensitivity variations in normal individuals, various factors, such as allergies, irritation, or anxiety, may produce a wide spectrum of readings in the Schirmer test. If one uses very low cutoff values, such as 3 mm of wetting in 5 minutes, the specificity (detection of normal eyes) of the test will be very high; however, the sensitivity in detecting persons with dry eyes will be low.

## Rose Bengal Staining

In the rose bengal staining test, the physician instills a red vegetable dye on the surface of the eye that stains cells that have lost their mucin coating (Figure 6). After the dye is placed on the eye's surface and allowed to rinse over the surface of the eye, the sides and central portion of the exposed eye are scored on a 0–3 scale for intensity of staining. The scores for three areas are added together. The cutoff for a dry eye is a minimum score of 3–5.

This test is very specific for dry eyes, but is not very sensitive. It frequently provides normal values in mild forms of dry eye, thus producing a false-negative result.

Rose bengal can cause stinging and irritation, especially when the eyes are dry. It is helpful if the physician rinses it out after the test is completed.

### Lysozyme and Lactoferrin

Dry eye patients have decreased lysozyme, an enzyme (type of protein). The lysozyme test measures the amount of lysozyme in tears. When compared with a group of normal patients, there is considerable overlap of values, so it is difficult to be sure to which group an individual patient belongs. Moreover, the test is difficult to perform and is not useful to individual patients.

Lactoferrin is a more stable antibacterial enzyme in tears, which can now be measured with a new, easily performed test. The consistently reliable readings obtained in normal patients indicate that this may be a good test for dry eye.

### Tear Osmolarity Test

The tear osmolarity test measures the particle concentration in tear film. For proper functioning, body fluids normally contain a certain concentration of salt. Tear osmolarity is a measure of this concentration, which in dry eye patients is hypertonic (higher than normal).

A tiny amount of tear fluid is drawn and specially prepared for analysis. Because the test was developed to measure resting tears and to avoid contamination by reflex tears that are present in so many other tests for dry eye, tear osmolarity appears to be more sensitive and specific than other tests.

Presently, tear osmolarity is available as a diagnostic test in only a few centers. Its advantage over other tests is that it gives more accurate, quantitative information about the degree of dryness in the eyes.

### Fluorescein Staining

Fluorescein is a vegetable dye that indicates points on the surface cells of the cornea that have rubbed off because of dryness. The dye is applied in a strip, which is moistened by touching the inside of the lower eyelid before the strip is instilled into the tears.

### Breakup Time

Fluorescein is also useful in staining tears to detect how well the cornea remains continuously covered with a tear film. Breakup time tests how well the cornea remains moistened between blinks. After a filter paper strip containing fluorescein is moistened with a nonpreserved saline solution, the fluorescein is instilled into the tears. Next, the patient blinks and then holds the eyes open for 10 seconds. A value of less than 10 seconds indicates a dry eye state.

## How Much Do These Tests Cost?

The cost of these tests varies widely by locality, by complexity, by the cost of materials and time, and by the physician's expertise. In many cases, the Schirmer test may be done merely as an addition to the regular eye examination. The tear osmolarity test, on the other hand, requires a technician and very precise electronic equipment. As a result, tear osmolarity is the most expensive test, requiring an additional fee.

## First Symptoms of Dry Eye

The symptoms of dry eye can vary considerably. Not only is the eye affected by abnormal tear composition, it is also sensitive to environmental agents such as low humidity, dust, and smoke. Its small size and small tear volume make it sensitive to evaporation. Fortunately, corneal nerve endings warn the individual when the eye is becoming dry. Only in certain neurological disorders, in which sensation and lid blinking are disturbed, is the eye likely to become dry without the patient's awareness. In addition to dryness, redness of the eye is likely to develop, as well as blurred vision. One of these three symptoms is usually sufficient to warn the patient and lead to a visit to an ophthalmologist.

## Treatments for Dry Eye

Current treatments are numerous, ranging from artificial tear solutions to plugging of the lacrimal puncta, the entrance to the drainage system for tears. Treating ocular dryness is an important medical issue. New therapies under development are moving rapidly to general availability.

### Artificial Tears

Artificial tears are made with and without preservatives. Some of the preservatives originally used were toxic, particularly if they were used more than six times a day. Many of the preservatives now used produce little or no toxicity. Artificial teardrops used frequently may also rinse away the normal tears needed to reestablish a normal tear film. Preservative-free solutions are prone to bacterial contamination; thus, they are frequently packaged in single-dose vials. The vial should be discarded after use in one or both eyes. Preservative-free solutions with different thicknesses or viscosities are available. For example, carboxymethylcellulose can be found in a 1.0 percent and a 0.5 percent solution. Recent additions to single-dose dry eye therapies include polycarbophil and a tear substitute that contains bicarbonate and simulates the natural tear film.

Although many dry eye patients use ointments, particularly at bedtime, some feel that ointments dry out in the eye, increasing the foreign body sensation. Others believe that ointments cause blurred vision on awakening.

Artificial tears primarily increase comfort. If the solution makes the patient more uncomfortable or burns, it is probably creating a toxic or sensitivity reaction. Another brand of artificial tears should be used instead.

### Hydroxypropyl Methylcellulose

Hydroxypropyl methylcellulose is available as a small chemical polymer rod that absorbs water and slowly dissolves, producing a film over normal tears. The film conserves tears by preventing evaporation. Unfortunately, many patients have difficulty inserting the very small pellet beneath the lower eyelid. Many patients also have an increased foreign body sensation after insertion. Artificial tears must be used with the pellet to supplement it and help it dissolve. For patients with mild to moderate dry eyes, the pellet often provides increased comfort.

### Moisture Chamber Glasses

Moisture chamber glasses are extremely helpful in conserving the small volume of tears in dry eye patients. Used in addition to tear substitutes, these custom-made eyeglasses also protect the eyes from exposure to air currents, such as air conditioning and wind gusts, and are helpful during long automobile and airplane trips. Swim goggles can also be used to seal in moisture; they are easily found in sporting goods stores.

## Punctal Occlusion

Punctal occlusion (closure of the tear ducts to provide an increased volume of tears by decreasing drainage) is accomplished in several ways. Whatever method is used, the lower puncta are usually sealed because they carry away the vast majority of the tears. Depending on subsequent improvement in symptoms, the upper puncta may be sealed later.

There are two types of punctal plugs, collagen and silicone. The collagen plug lasts only a short time, may not occlude completely, and is eventually absorbed. This can help both the patient and the physician evaluate the value of punctal occlusion.

The silicone plug is not absorbed and can be removed easily. This is important. If the patient's condition improves and tears are once again produced in greater amounts, the plug will no longer be needed.

Just as connective tissue diseases vary, a dry eye condition can vary in severity. Fluctuation in tear production is not uncommon in patients who are believed to be in the early stages of Sjogren's syndrome.

As a permanent treatment, the puncta can be closed surgically by electrocautery or argon laser. Surgical occlusion may have to be repeated since the puncta tend to reopen. On the other hand, once they are closed, they are difficult to reopen. For this reason, temporary or semipermanent punctal occlusion may be performed by the ophthalmologist using cautery or the laser. If it is beneficial, a more permanent procedure can be performed.

## Vitamin A Ointment

Current studies indicate that vitamin A ointment (tretinoin) may be helpful for a few patients with relatively rare, severe dry eye conditions.

## Common Treatment Problems

After starting artificial tear therapy, many patients are disappointed. They may expect a complete cure or become tired of repeatedly instilling artificial tears to obtain relief. Like many skin conditions, the dry eye is frequently helped by medication but hardly ever completely cured.

To become efficient and avoid drenching the face, instilling artificial tears takes practice. Excessive drops on the lashes should be removed with a clean tissue or cotton pad since rapid drying on the lid margin may lead to flakes, which can irritate the eye. Allergies to pollen and animal dander can add to eye irritation in persons with dry eyes. Also, certain artificial tears, especially those with a high preservative content, can be irritating.

Tap water should never be instilled into the eye because even the best city water supplies may contain bacteria. Any solution instilled into the eye must be sterile and, if free of preservatives, used no later than 36 hours after opening. Even a sterile solution should not be kept for more than 3 months once the bottle is opened.

Lid hygiene will make the patient more comfortable. Warm compresses soften dried secretions from the lid margin, which then can be removed with a dry Q-Tip.

General body hygiene, with the use of shampoo and soap containing antibacterial compounds, is important to decrease the number of bacteria on the skin. Bacteria entering a dry eye with decreased local resistance may cause infections. Rubbing the eyes with soiled tissues or dirty fingers is asking for trouble.

Having the eyes examined periodically by doctors, following their advice, and using medications properly will prevent damage to vision and usually provide maximum comfort.

### Cataract Surgery in Dry Eye Patients

Dry eye patients undergoing cataract surgery can expect slightly greater irritation and a slightly longer visual recovery period. Fortunately, dry eye is superficial and usually does not interfere with wound healing. Continued treatment of the dry eye during the recovery period is sometimes necessary, in spite of increased stimulation of reflex tears by the operative wound.

### Blepharitis

Blepharitis (inflammation of the eyelids) is commonly associated with dry eye. It frequently requires treatment in addition to dry eye treatments. Blepharitis may arise from several factors but appears related primarily to the secretions from the numerous meibomian glands in the eyelid, which are released through openings in the upper and lower margins. In blepharitis, the secretions appear excessive and seem to clog the openings on the lid margin, leading to reddened lid margins, crusts, granulations, small ulcers, styes, and chalazion (a small bump) on the eyelid margin.

Blepharitis causes constant and severe discomfort, not only because of the lid disease but also because of the accompanying dry eye, which apparently results from abnormalities in the lipid layer of the tear film. This condition is treated by applying warm compresses to the lids, using tap water and an ordinary washcloth. Heat on the lid for 5 to 10 minutes, depending on the severity of the blepharitis, softens the lipid secretions of the lid, so that they can be removed more easily from the lid and gland openings. After removing the warm compresses, the patient should firmly massage the lid margins behind the eyelashes with a clean finger. Many ophthalmologists prescribe an oral antibiotic, doxycycline, for a few months to treat blepharitis.

Some physicians recommend using baby shampoo or special soaps and pads to cleanse the lids. Patients should use what works best for them. One approach is to make the routine as simple as possible, similar to chores like brushing and flossing the teeth after every meal. Frequently, these are not done by persons in a rush to do other things that seem more important. Baby shampoo used on the eyelid, however, particularly if one has trouble keeping the shampoo confined to the lid margin, may get into the tear film, where it will interfere with tear film function.

Many patients with blepharitis often ask whether this condition will ever disappear or whether they will have to perform lid hygiene indefinitely. Since blepharitis is more of a skin condition than a disease, it will probably remain indefinitely to some degree, depending on many factors such as perspiration and gland secretion.

Eye rubbing with unwashed fingers and inadequate removal of oils, makeup, and secretions will make blepharitis worse. Regular lid hygiene not only decreases blepharitis by preventing inflammation and symptoms of dry eye, it also prevents infections of the eyelids, such as styes and lid ulcerations. Regular attention to cleaning the lid margins illustrates the adage that "An ounce of prevention is worth a pound of cure."

## Activities and Conditions That Aggravate the Eye

- Reading, studying, and/or prolonged work at a computer terminal decrease the blink rate. Try blinking on purpose.
- Low humidity
- Air conditioning
- Air currents

- Dust and fumes

- Smoke

- Excessive makeup, especially on the eyelid margin. Makeup is all right as long as it is kept mainly on the tips of the eyelashes and the skin of the lid. If it is applied too close to the base of the eyelashes, it tends to soften and run, allowing it to enter the tear film and result in more concentrated tears

- Parasympathetic drugs that make the mouth dry, such as tranquilizers, antihistamines, and diuretics.

### Directions for the Future

It is heartening to note that researchers are always looking for ways to improve the treatment of dry eyes. Several approaches are under investigation. With certain treatments, the benefits are obvious to the patient and physician when they are being tested. With others, years of study may be required before we know if they will or will not work. This section deals with some of the new innovations in the treatment of dry eyes.

### Pilocarpine

Pilocarpine is a plant-derived substance that affects nerve endings and the transmission of impulses across nerves. In large doses, it can stimulate secretory glands such as the salivary and lacrimal glands. Its main use is as an eye drop in the treatment of glaucoma. In fact, it was the first-line treatment for glaucoma until the late 1970s. Recently, an oral form of pilocarpine was approved for the treatment of dry mouth. Studies are underway at several medical centers to determine its effect on dry eyes. While the results so far seem encouraging, pilocarpine has some systemic side effects such as nausea, sweating, headaches, frequent urination, and diarrhea. Most individuals tolerate oral pilocarpine quite well.

### New Formulations of Artificial Tears

Researchers and pharmaceutical companies are constantly striving to make better artificial tears. Most would like to have a preparation that is effective for a long time and does not cause blurring or other side effects. One approach is to develop tear formulations that mimic the normal tear composition. One product has an electrolyte composition very close to that of normal tears. Unlike other artificial tears, it contains bicarbonate, a component of normal tears. Because bicarbonate is unstable, special packaging is required. Another product employs a viscous droplet that is instilled into the eye and acts as a reservoir, replenishing the tear film for a sustained period of time. A tear gel has been available in Europe for some time, and a similar product is under investigation in the United States. Yet another product was designed to maintain the health of the ocular surface by a unique electrolyte composition and hypotonicity. Other attempts to devise a beneficial artificial tear include the use of sodium hyaluronate, a substance commonly used in eye surgery. In its present form, it is expensive and has to be diluted by the practitioner or a cooperative pharmacist. Some doctors and patients find this drop quite useful. Collagen, a key component of skin and other tissues, can be broken down into small pieces and combined with a lipid to form a substance known as lacrisomes. In some preliminary studies, people with dry eyes find lacrisomes to be soothing and long-lasting.

## Cyclosporine

Several years ago, researchers noted that cyclosporine, a drug used to prevent transplant rejection, increased tear secretion in dogs with dry eyes due to a variety of causes. It is thought that cyclosporine stimulates a receptor on lacrimal gland secretory cells. Cyclosporine eye drops are now being tested in dry eye patients.

## Vitamin A

Vitamin A and related preparations have a theoretical role in the treatment of dry eye. Vitamin A maintains the moisture of mucosal surfaces, whereas vitamin A–deficient individuals develop dry eye and a drying out of the ocular surface. Early clinical trials with vitamin A drops and ointment were encouraging, but further studies did not justify the early enthusiasm. It is possible that we will see further studies with vitamin A using different doses and methods of delivery to the eye.

## Hormones

The prevalence of dry eye in menopausal and postmenopausal women has raised the question of its possible association with hormone deficiency. It has been suggested that low levels of hormones, either estrogens or androgens, may affect tear production. Oral estrogens have been prescribed to treat a variety of postmenopausal problems. The effects of oral estrogens on dry eyes have not been striking; however, further research is required to determine if some type of hormonal therapy may be beneficial. Recently, it has been demonstrated that androgens support lacrimal secretion. Research is underway to define their effects further.

## Moisture Glasses

Special glasses have been devised in Japan that use small, wet sponges inserted on specially designed side panels to increase the humidity surrounding the eyes. The side panels hold the sponges and act as additional barriers to evaporation of tears. The sponges are replaced every 1–2 weeks. Although moisture glasses are not readily available in the United States, they seem to have helped many dry eye patients in Japan.

Troy E. Daniels, DDS, MS

Irwin D. Mandel, DDS

James J. Sciubba, DMD, PhD

# 6 Salivary and Oral Conditions

SALIVA IS ONE of our natural resources. Too often the bounty of a natural resource is not appreciated until there is a shortage.

Patients with Sjogren's syndrome have different amounts of reduction in saliva flow. However, in all but the most severe cases, there is some increase in this flow following stimulation with taste or chewing. In many patients, however, there is little saliva flow without stimulation.

People with Sjogren's syndrome may also have other diseases that require the long-term use of medication for treatment. Many of these medications can reduce salivary flow as a side effect, thus compounding the patient's problem. Since saliva is a complex fluid containing a variety of components and serving many physiological needs, a marked shortage of this fluid can produce discomfort; impair oral function in chewing, swallowing, and speaking; and lead to damage to the teeth and oral mucous membranes.

Saliva is produced by three pairs of major salivary glands: the parotid glands, located in front of the ears; the submandibular glands, located between the lower jaw and the base of the tongue; and the sublingual glands, located in the floor of the mouth, under the tongue. These major glands produce about 95 percent of the saliva. The rest comes from numerous pinhead-size minor salivary glands located in many areas inside the mouth, just beneath the surface. These minor glands are especially numerous in the areas of the lips and palate. In patients with Sjogren's syndrome, both the major and minor glands are affected. These patients have very different levels of salivary dysfunction and intensity of symptoms.

There are three very different rates of salivary secretion, normally or in patients with Sjogren's syndrome. Maximum secretion occurs when we are tasting, chewing, or smelling something (called stimulated flow). The second rate occurs during most of our waking hours, when we produce saliva much more slowly than during stimulation (called resting flow). The lowest rate occurs during sleep, when very little saliva is produced (less than one-tenth as much as resting flow). Patients with Sjogren's syndrome usually have reductions in all three of these rates.

### Specific Functions of Saliva

A brief discussion of the specific function of saliva will clarify how and why oral problems occur when there is not enough saliva.

Contrary to common belief, the main function of saliva is not to digest starches. Saliva does indeed contain a large amount of the enzyme amylase, which digests starch, but the pancreas also produces a great deal of amylase. The amount of salivary amylase is not critical to digestion.

When we ingest and digest food, salivary secretions mainly aid in chewing, swallowing, and tasting. The mucus component of saliva covers the food bolus which helps it move along the chewing and swallowing surfaces. The water and other components of saliva provide the appropriate environment for the taste buds to function.

Since we are not eating most of the time, the salivary glands are not being stimulated by taste or chewing stimuli. Yet the small amount of resting salivary flow helps to maintain the structure of the teeth and mucous membranes of the mouth and throat. The combined saliva from the major and minor glands contains a variety of salts, proteins, carbohydrates (starch and sugar), and lipids (fats), which give it considerable protective properties.

Saliva has five major protective functions:

1   *Coating and lubricating the mucous membranes*. In addition to covering the food bolus, the salivary mucins stick to and coat all the tissues of the mouth. This produces the smooth sensation one normally feels when the tongue passes over the lips, teeth, or gums. The mucin coating serves as a natural barrier to irritating com-

ponents in food and beverages, as well as to toxic products generated by bacteria in the mouth and to the drying effect of mouth breathing. This coating on the teeth and soft tissues also allows ready passage of the food bolus and enables the teeth to glide smoothly over each other during chewing.

2 *Mechanical cleansing.* The flow of saliva and the muscle activity of the lips and tongue remove most food remnants and large numbers of potentially harmful bacteria from the teeth and soft tissues. The maximal effect occurs during eating, when the combination of taste and chewing stimulation produces the maximal flow of saliva. This clearance mechanism is similar to tearing and blinking in the eye, blowing the nose, and coughing to clear the lungs.

3 *Maintenance of neutrality.* Saliva contains components that buffer and neutralize acidic and basic (alkaline) foods and beverages, helping to keep the oral cavity chemically neutral (pH of 7.0). If the oral environment is too acidic or too basic, the soft and hard tissues in the mouth can be injured. Saliva influences acid formation in the bacterial plaques (thin films) that form on tooth surfaces. These plaques can convert the various kinds of sugar in the diet into acids that begin the process of tooth decay. Normal salivary flow provides a continuous source of buffering substances that helps to neutralize the acids as they are formed.

4 *Maintenance of tooth structure.* Teeth are made up of a crystalline substance, composed mainly of calcium and phosphate in a special configuration, called hydroxyapatite. To prevent dissolution of these crystals, normal saliva contains an appropriate concentration of calcium and phosphate salts, kept in balance by specialized proteins. In the absence or severe reduction of saliva, this balance between the calcium and phosphate in the tooth and in the saliva is disturbed, and teeth are more susceptible to decay or erosion by acidic foods and beverages. The mucin coating on the teeth described above also protects against erosion, abrasion, and physical wear.

5 *Antibacterial activity.* In addition to physically removing bacteria, saliva can affect bacteria in other ways. Coating of bacteria by mucin and other salivary proteins causes clumping of the bacteria, so that they cannot stick to teeth or soft tissues and are swallowed. A special

antibody in saliva, called secretory IgA, can also coat oral bacteria, preventing their attachment to teeth or soft tissues. A group of salivary proteins (lysozyme, lactoferrin, peroxidase, and histatins), working in conjunction with other components of saliva, can have an immediate effect on oral bacteria, interfering with their ability to multiply or killing them directly. Protective components in saliva can also be effective against yeast cells (*Candida*) and viruses, including the virus associated with acquired immunodeficiency syndrome (AIDS).

## Clinical Features

Some or all of the following clinical features are seen in most patients with Sjogren's syndrome with widely different levels of severity. However, they are not unique to Sjogren's syndrome and may also be seen in patients who have other conditions associated with significant reductions in the quantity of saliva produced, or as a result of treatment of coexisting medical conditions.

### Symptoms (Changes Patients Feel)

The principal oral symptom of Sjogren's syndrome is a feeling of dryness, sometimes called xerostomia. However, not all patients describe their problem this way. Some may mention difficulty in swallowing food, problems in wearing complete dentures, changes in the sense of taste, discomfort and/or burning symptoms in the mouth, or inability to eat dry foods. These symptoms usually develop very gradually. In some patients, their severity may fluctuate slowly over weeks or months.

### Signs (Changes That Can Be Seen or Palpated)

Following are the various clinical signs that may be seen in patients with Sjogren's syndrome:

- *Major salivary glands.* The parotid or submandibular glands in Sjogren's syndrome may show various degrees of firm enlargement, usually without pain or tenderness. About one-third of patients with Sjogren's syndrome will develop this enlargement in their major salivary glands at some time. Many Sjogren's syndrome patients with major salivary gland enlargement report that it occurs in episodes lasting for many weeks or months, while other patients have chronic enlargement with very slow changes in size. The swelling may begin on one side of the face but eventually affects both sides.

- *Oral signs.* (1) Dry, sticky oral mucosal surfaces; (2) dental caries (tooth decay), primarily affecting the teeth at the gum line or on the incisal edges of the front teeth; (3) cloudy, thickened saliva or no saliva expressible from the parotid or submandibular ducts; (4) smooth or cobblestone appearance of the tongue, with or without fissures; (5) areas of redness on the roof of the mouth, inside the cheeks, under dentures, or on the tongue; and (6) angular cheilitis (sores at the corners of the mouth). Signs (4), (5), and (6) are usually associated with the symptom of burning and are usually caused by candidiasis, which is described below.

### Dental Caries (Tooth Decay)

One of the earliest and most common oral problems in patients with Sjogren's syndrome is increased tooth decay, which may be rapidly progressive. The marked reduction in saliva volume, along with the loss of its protective and antibacterial properties, results in increased retention of bacterial plaque and food debris around the teeth, especially at the gum line. With a reduction in salivary flow, the saliva becomes more acidic. A less protective, more acidic saliva causes a change in the balance of various bacterial organisms that make up the dental plaque. Organisms that live well in such an environment thrive at the expense of their neighbors. *Streptococcus mutans*, the bacterium with the greatest potential for producing decay, increases rapidly in number.

To compound this problem, when many people first experience symptoms of dry mouth, they often use sucrose (sugar)-containing candies or gum to stimulate the flow of saliva. However, sugar provides bacteria in the dental plaque with an ideal substance for producing destructive acids on the tooth surfaces. Sugar-containing snacks lead rapidly to decay; they must not be used. Instead, nonsucrose sweeteners such as sorbitol, xylitol, or aspartame should be used.

In persons with dry mouth, the most decay-prone part of the tooth is at the gum line. In older individuals who have recessed gums, the exposed cementum or dentin can be attacked very rapidly, resulting in root caries (tooth decay near or under the gum tissue). Tooth enamel is also susceptible, especially at the margins of old fillings, where there may be chips, breaks, and roughness. "My fillings are falling out" is a common complaint. The junctions of tooth surfaces with gold, plastic, or porcelain crowns (caps) are particularly vulnerable to tooth decay. In the severely dry mouth, however, all surfaces are at risk, even those not usually susceptible to decay, such as the biting edges of the incisor teeth.

### Tooth Erosion and Abrasion

In addition to tooth decay, tooth structure can be lost by the direct attack of acids contained in foods, beverages, and confections, as well as by abrasion due to physical forces. Excessive use of citrus fruits or frequent use of very sour candies should be avoided. Moderation is the key. Soft drinks, which are very acidic, should be ingested with a straw to bypass the teeth and should not contain sucrose. The teeth should be brushed with a soft toothbrush, with light pressure and a fluoride-containing toothpaste. Overly abrasive toothpastes (those designed for smokers or persons with heavy tooth stains) should be avoided.

### Gingivitis and Periodontitis

The increased retention of plaque on the teeth next to the gum can result in gingivitis (inflammation of the gums). This is controllable with good oral hygiene. However, there is no evidence that the more serious form of periodontal disease, periodontitis (inflammation of the tissues surrounding and supporting the teeth), is increased in patients with Sjogren's syndrome.

### Soft Tissues

In many patients with decreased saliva, the oral mucosa may become red, smooth, and shiny, and it may be dry and sticky when touched. The upper surface of the tongue is usually the first area to show such a change. Its appearance may range from slight reddening, with loss of the normal carpet-like texture, to a deep red color and a cobblestone texture. There may be painless grooves on the tongue's surface. These signs are often associated with the symptom of burning and with the patient's growing intolerance of acidic or spicy foods. These changes are usually caused by candidiasis, which is described below. Patients wearing complete dentures have special difficulties. The lack of adequate saliva may allow the tongue to stick to dentures, especially the lower one, causing it to shift when chewing and swallowing, and leading to sore spots and ulcerations on the soft tissue.

### Candidiasis

In this condition, the yeast *Candida* overgrows and causes a superficial infection and thinning of the soft tissue lining the mouth. *Candida* species are normal inhabitants of most mouths in very small numbers, but conditions such as Sjogren's syndrome can cause them to proliferate. With a reduced quantity and quality of saliva and resulting changes in the chemical and physical nature of the oral environment, *Candida* can grow in great numbers.

An early sign of candidiasis is white patches on the tongue, cheeks, or palate, but most frequently the affected mucosa appears red, with symptoms of burning or tenderness. Areas covered by a complete denture are often affected. Specific antifungal drugs are required to treat this condition, as described below. Even with effective initial treatment, however, this overgrowth often recurs and must be retreated.

### Miscellaneous Problems

In some patients, a variety of other oral disturbances can occur, including difficulties in swallowing, oral malodor, changes in the sense of taste, intolerance of acidic or spicy foods, or difficulty in recognizing the normal taste of specific foods. These problems may lessen or resolve with adequate treatment of oral candidiasis. Swallowing is difficult because of an inadequate mucin coating on the food bolus and oral mucosa, which interferes with the smooth movement of the food from the back of the mouth to the esophagus. Constant sipping of water during meals may be necessary. Oral malodor can arise from retention of food remnants in the mouth and overgrowth of certain bacteria, especially on the tongue; careful oral hygiene is essential.

## Diagnosis of Oral Problems in Sjogren's Syndrome

Sjogren's syndrome needs to be diagnosed early so that damage to the teeth and eyes can be prevented. But the diagnosis must be made carefully to distinguish between the various causes of dry eye and dry mouth symptoms and signs. Because Sjogren's syndrome is chronic in all patients and progressive in some, an incorrect diagnosis can cause a

---

**TABLE 5   CAUSES OF DECREASED SALIVARY SECRETION**

---

*Temporary*

    Effects of short-term drug use (e.g., antihistamines)
    Viral and bacterial infections (e.g., mumps)
    Dehydration
    Psychological causes (e.g., fear, depression)

*Chronic*

    Effects of many chronically administered drugs (e.g., many of those used to treat depression,
      high blood pressure, allergies, Parkinson's disease, or psychiatric conditions)
    Systemic diseases
      Sjogren's syndrome
      Granulomatous diseases (sarcoidosis, tuberculosis, leprosy)
      Amyloidosis
      Human immunodeficiency virus infection
      Graft-versus-host disease
      Cystic fibrosis
      Diabetes mellitus (uncontrolled)
    Therapeutic radiation of the head and neck
    Trauma or surgery of the head and neck

---

patient years of unnecessary concern about his or her health. No one test will establish the presence of Sjogren's syndrome. Therefore, each component (salivary, ocular, and systemic) is diagnosed separately. At least two of these three components must be established by reliable, objective diagnostic criteria for Sjogren's syndrome to be confirmed.

Although dry mouth is part of most definitions of Sjogren's syndrome and is certainly an important problem for most patients, it should not be used to diagnose the salivary component of Sjogren's syndrome. Symptoms of dry mouth are interpreted differently by the patient experiencing them, and dry mouth can be caused by a variety of conditions in addition to Sjogren's syndrome (Table 5). Most often, dry mouth symptoms are caused by prescription drugs.

The means of assessing salivary glands include measuring saliva production, x-ray examination of the glands, nuclear medicine examination, measuring components of saliva, and salivary gland biopsy. All these methods have a role in the diagnosis of various salivary gland diseases, but they are not equally helpful in diagnosing the salivary component of Sjogren's syndrome.

## Measuring Saliva Production

Salivary flow rates can be measured for whole saliva (from all the glands) or for parotid or submandibular gland secretions separately, either unstimulated or stimulated by taste or chewing. Unstimulated whole salivary flow rates measure a patient's basal or resting salivary secretion. These rates, which are reduced in Sjogren's syndrome, most closely reflect a patient's symptoms of dry mouth. But they are also reduced as a side effect of many commonly prescribed drugs and by diseases other than Sjogren's syndrome.

Separate flow rates from parotid or submandibular glands, measured with taste or chewing stimulation, give an estimate of the amount of saliva the gland can secrete on demand. However, these rates are proportional to the size of the gland, which varies among individuals. Standardized measurements of stimulated salivary flow are useful in determining an individual's salivary gland function and offer a noninvasive way to follow an individual's course of a chronic disease such as Sjogren's syndrome. However, they also may be reduced by diseases other than Sjogren's syndrome. Salivary flow rates exhibit such a wide range of variation among individuals without disease that no value can provide a reliable distinction between normal and abnormal flow.

## X-Ray Examination

Sialography is a method for examining changes in the duct system of the major salivary glands. A liquid contrast medium (a substance visible by x-ray) is injected slowly into the salivary gland through its duct opening in the mouth. This method is still used to examine patients with Sjogren's syndrome, but it has some important limitations: The changes revealed by this test are not specific to Sjogren's syndrome; some types of x-ray contrast media used in this technique can cause unacceptable side effects; and safer contrast media are less effective in detecting changes in the ducts. This procedure is giving way to better methods and is used infrequently.

## Nuclear Medicine Examination

Sequential salivary scintigraphy is a diagnostic technique involving injection of a tiny quantity of low-level radioactive material into a vein. The radioactive material soon localizes in the major salivary glands. It is detected by examining the head and neck with a special sensitive camera that can locate the radioactive material. This can be used to assess the metabolic function of the major salivary glands simultaneously.

In Sjogren's syndrome patients, uptake of the radioactive material by the glands and the appearance of radioactive saliva in the mouth are delayed or absent. Salivary scintigraphic findings correlate with stimulated parotid flow rate measurements, but these findings are not diagnostically specific for Sjogren's syndrome.

### Measuring Salivary Components

Measuring the amount of various chemical or immunological constituents in saliva is called sialochemistry. In several studies with Sjogren's syndrome patients, these measurements have shown some promise for aiding our understanding of the salivary component of this disease and may be helpful in following disease progression. However, they are not specific enough to serve as diagnostic tests for Sjogren's syndrome, and they are not widely available.

### Salivary Gland Biopsy

Labial salivary gland biopsy (microscopically examining minor salivary glands from the inside of the lower lip) offers the most disease-specific way to diagnose the salivary component of Sjogren's syndrome. The microscope can reveal the characteristic process of Sjogren's syndrome, a distinctive pattern of infiltration of the affected glands by lymphocytes (a type of white blood cell). These infiltrates are similar to those seen in any of the organs affected by Sjogren's syndrome, including the salivary glands, lacrimal (tear) glands, liver, kidney, and lungs. The infiltrates cause the affected organs to function abnormally, producing such symptoms as dry mouth or dry eyes.

Because Sjogren's syndrome is a systemic disease, it affects both major and minor salivary glands. Biopsy of minor glands avoids the need to biopsy a major gland, usually the parotid, which can produce facial scarring, possible nerve damage, and salivary fistula formation (abnormal drainage of saliva through the skin of the face). Recent studies have described safer ways to biopsy the parotid gland. However, these biopsy specimens are generally less satisfactory for diagnosing the salivary component of Sjogren's syndrome than specimens from labial glands, especially for patients with early or mild Sjogren's syndrome.

Labial salivary gland biopsy involves removal of several pinhead-size minor glands under local anesthesia from the inside of the lower lip. Performed as an outpatient procedure, the salivary gland biopsy can reveal the characteristic infiltration pattern of Sjogren's syndrome. The biopsy will not make the patient's dry mouth worse. In the absence of Sjogren's syndrome, the biopsy may reveal other causes of dry mouth.

## Treating Dry Mouth

While Sjogren's syndrome is not curable, the oral problems are manageable. Treatment can reduce the patient's symptoms and prevent or reduce irreversible damage to the teeth and eyes. The goals in managing the salivary component of Sjogren's syndrome include (1) preventing and treating dental caries; (2) diagnosing and treating oral candidiasis; (3) stimulating salivary flow; (4) selectively using saliva substitutes; and (5) possibly making changes in prescription drug use. Each of these goals is described in Chapter 21.

# 7 Ear, Nose, and Throat Problems

*Although the world is full of suffering, it is also full of the over-coming of it.* —*Helen Keller*

GRITTY EYES. A dry, sore, sticky mouth and throat. A husky voice. A stopped-up, scabby, bloody nose. A diminished sense of smell and taste. Stuffy ears. Painful joints. To Sjogren's syndrome patients, these symptoms may seem as awful as the plagues called down on Pharaoh by Moses, and may rob those who suffer from them of many of the comforts of life and the enjoyment of living.

Sjogren's syndrome affects more than the salivary and lacrimal (tear) glands and the joints. The mouth, pharynx (throat), larynx (voice box), nose, and ears are affected by dryness, too. Several parts of the body may suffer as the autoimmune process progresses, gradually destroying the parotid, submandibular, and sublingual (major salivary) glands; drying up the hundreds of minor salivary glands in the lips, mouth, and throat; and depriving the larynx and ears of needed moisture.

## How Is the Mouth Affected?

As the salivary glands lose their ability to produce saliva, the individual will experience xerostomia (dry mouth), often accompanied by burning and soreness. Constant thirst is a common complaint. Fissures (cracks) may develop at the corners of the lips as they become irritated and raw from the lack of moisture. The tongue may become red or lumpy. Dental caries (tooth decay) may be rampant, and difficulty in retaining dentures becomes evident. (The effects of Sjogren's syndrome on the teeth and other oral components of Sjogren's syndrome are discussed in Chapter 6.)

People with xerostomia are more likely to have oral candidiasis (a yeast-like fungal infection, such as thrush). This causes even more soreness and burning, red oral membranes, and, occasionally, white patches. Affected individuals may notice loss of the sense of taste, partly because the membranes in the mouth are dry and partly because dryness disrupts taste bud architecture and function.

## How Is the Nose Affected?

The thousands of tiny mucous glands in all areas of the nose are also damaged in Sjogren's syndrome. Nasal functions include cleansing and humidification of the air breathed. With dryness, the nose becomes congested and stuffy. As the dry crusts detach from the nasal membranes, occasional bleeding may occur. Although annoying, the bleeding is rarely severe. The drier and crustier the nose becomes, the less acute is the sense of smell.

## How Are the Ears Affected?

Just as Sjogren's syndrome damages the moisture-producing glands of the mouth and nose, it may also injure the mucous glands of the eustachian tube (the tube running from the back of the nose to the middle ear). When this occurs, the ears may feel stuffy, and hearing acuity decreases. If mucous glands within the middle ear itself become involved, middle ear infections may result. Fortunately, this does not happen very often in Sjogren's syndrome patients.

Autoimmune diseases have been associated with inner ear pathology. Fortunately, this is very uncommon in primary Sjogren's syndrome; however, rheumatoid arthritis, which is a common problem in secondary Sjogren's syndrome, has been associated with both middle ear (mechanical or conductive) hearing loss and inner ear (nerve) hearing loss.

Hearing loss has so many possible causes, especially prior infection, excessive noise exposure, and aging, that Sjogren's syndrome patients should not jump to the conclusion that a hearing or balance problem is due to their autoimmune condition. However, if none of the above risk factors are present, then it would be appropriate to ask pertinent questions of both an ear specialist and a rheumatologist.

## How Is the Larynx Affected?

Mucous glands within the larynx are necessary for speaking. If the autoimmune disease causes these glands to atrophy, the surface of the vocal cords will become dry, and thick clusters of mucus may stick to them. The voice will become husky, and the patient may have to constantly clear the throat to dislodge the mucus. Dealing with voice problems is thoroughly discussed in Chapter 22.

## How Are the Salivary Glands Affected?

Often the first and most common symptom of Sjogren's syndrome is discomfort due to swelling of the major salivary glands. The swelling is caused by infiltration of these glands by lymphocytes. Although these glands rarely become infected in Sjogren's syndrome, when they do, swelling is rapid and painful, accompanied by tenderness, fever, and possibly redness.

## Tests for Sjogren's Syndrome

Some would argue that because the diagnosis of Sjogren's syndrome can be made so readily on the basis of symptoms, diagnostic tests are unnecessary. Others ask: "Why bother testing patients who have dry eyes, dry mouth, swollen salivary glands, and rheumatoid arthritis? What else could it be but Sjogren's syndrome? And you're not going to treat these patients anyway."

But other diseases, such as sarcoidosis and tuberculosis, may cause the same symptoms. These treatable disorders must be ruled out or managed. Moreover, as Sjogren's syndrome advances and becomes more troublesome, antimetabolite (cyclophosphamide or methotrexate, for example) and/or steroid therapy may help. These therapies cannot be offered without a biopsy or blood tests to support the diagnosis of Sjogren's syndrome.

The following four tests may be performed or ordered by the otolaryngologist in evaluating a possible case of Sjogren's syndrome: (1) lip biopsy, (2) sialography, (3) salivary gland scan, and (4) salivary flow rate. These tests are discussed in detail in Chapters 4 and 6.

## Prescription Treatments That Stimulate Saliva and Mucus

Unlike over-the-counter remedies that alleviate the symptoms of dryness, prescribed treatments are designed to stimulate saliva and mucus production. Despite destruction of the secretory elements in the moisture-producing glands, enough function may remain to benefit from some form of stimulation. Other medical conditions may make the use of any of these prescription drugs inappropriate.

Systemic (bodywide) iodides, prescribed as potassium iodide, help promote nasal and throat secretions. They are usually quite safe. Their side effects, however, include iodine allergy and stomach upset.

Pilocarpine is an effective stimulant of both the mucous and salivary glands and may be used either topically in the nose or taken by mouth. Because the range between efficacy and toxicity is narrow, this drug must be used under close medical supervision. It is now available by prescription in an oral tablet that is taken three times daily. It has several side effects and is not appropriate for everybody (see Chapter 21).

Guaifenesin, the main ingredient in most expectorants, increases respiratory tract fluid and helps to loosen phlegm and mucus. It is also available in a more concentrated form, as are other medications that are available by only by prescription.

## Other Drugs That May Help or Harm

When nasal allergy is thought to be a problem, one of many nasal cortisone sprays (available by prescription only) may be very helpful. There are a host of medications that can clearly aggravate the dryness: antihistamines, decongestants, tranquilizers and other psychotropic drugs, some antihypertensive medications, diuretics, some antidiarrheal preparations, and many narcotics are the chief offenders. If a new medication is used and the dryness gets worse, the patient should be suspicious.

## Air Travel

Unfortunately, aircraft interiors are significantly drier than even most centrally heated homes. Together with the exceedingly poor ventilation systems on most airplanes, this very dry air can cause significant distress to the Sjogren's syndrome patient. When flying, the patient should keep the nasal membranes constantly moistened by spraying with saline solution. A glass of nonalcoholic fluid should be consumed every half hour.

# Extraglandular
## Involvement

**Harry Spiera, MD**

**Harry Moutsopoulos, MD**

# 8 Connective Tissue Disorders and Vasculitis

THE HALLMARK SYMPTOMS of Sjogren's syndrome, dry eyes or dry mouth, may also be accompanied by swollen, red, hot, tender joints; joint pain without swelling; muscle pain and weakness; skin rashes; or symptoms of major organ dysfunction. Patients with these additional symptoms may be diagnosed as having secondary Sjogren's syndrome. These patients may have one or more of the associated connective tissue diseases.

Connective tissue includes the various structural tissues that literally hold the various organs together. Bones, muscles, tendons, ligaments, and a component called ground substance are generally categorized as connective tissue. The connective tissue diseases most commonly associated with Sjogren's syndrome are rheumatoid arthritis, systemic lupus erythematosus, scleroderma, and dermatomyositis.

## Common Factors

The causes of all of these connective tissue diseases are unknown, but each manifests features of autoimmunity (a condition in which the immune system mistakenly attacks the body's own tissues). Our knowledge of autoimmune diseases is limited; clinicians and scientists are still describing these disorders. The physician's tools are knowledge about the disease patterns, the type of symptoms, the kinds of tissues involved, and some of the characteristic abnormalities in blood tests. These help the physician make a diagnosis.

All autoimmune diseases are chronic and unpredictable. The course

**71**

of the disease varies with each patient. Some patients may even improve spontaneously. Patients experience varying degrees of illness and disability. Sjogren's syndrome complicates the illness it accompanies. In some patients, Sjogren's syndrome itself becomes the cardinal problem.

The physician who cares for patients with various connective tissue diseases must be alert for the symptoms and manifestations of Sjogren's syndrome. While there are treatments for all of these diseases, cures have not yet been found. Treatments directed at Sjogren's syndrome, whether associated with a connective tissue disease or not, are discussed in other chapters of this book. They are not the same as treatments for the various connective tissue diseases described here.

### Rheumatoid Arthritis

Rheumatoid arthritis is mainly a disease of the joints. For unknown reasons, the joints become inflamed and painfully swollen, red, hot, and tender. Although any joint in the body may be involved, the metacarpophalangeal and proximal interphalangeal joints of the hands (knuckles), wrists, elbows, shoulders, knees, ankles, and feet are the ones usually affected by rheumatoid arthritis. Swelling and pain may subside, but a characteristic deformation of the joints may remain. Rheumatoid arthritis is a common disease afflicting approximately 1 percent of the population, women twice as frequently as men. It can occur at any age. An estimated 250,000 children in the United States alone have juvenile rheumatoid arthritis. At the other end of the age spectrum, patients in their nineties may suffer from an acute form of rheumatoid arthritis.

Although rheumatoid arthritis primarily involves joints, it is a generalized illness and can affect several organ systems. Many patients have anemia and fever and are easily fatigued. On occasion, rheumatoid arthritis may affect the heart, lungs, nerves, skin, and eyes. In a significant number of patients, the disease is associated with inflammation of salivary and lacrimal glands. These patients have secondary Sjogren's syndrome.

Rheumatoid arthritis is treated in several ways. For some patients, rest, a range-of-motion exercise program, and aspirin to relieve pain and swelling are sufficient treatment. However, if the disease becomes more severe or progressive, a physician may prescribe nonsteroidal anti-inflammatory agents or steroids (see Chapter 20).

In some cases, doctors use medicines that seem to have the capacity to modify the illness rather than just relieve symptoms. These medicines include methotrexate, gold, *d*-penicillamine, the antimalarial drugs (quinine derivatives first developed to treat malaria), and immunosuppressive agents. All of these medicines have potentially serious side effects. Their use must be monitored carefully by a physician well acquainted with the effects and side effects of these powerful drugs.

Cortisone, a well-known steroid very effective in reducing inflammation, and its derivatives, particularly prednisone, are often administered either by mouth or by injection directly into the joint to suppress pain, swelling, and inflammation. However, like all powerful medicines, cortisone also has potentially serious side effects. The physician and the patient must weigh the potential benefits against the potential risks for the individual course of treatment.

Physical therapy is often part of the treatment plan. This pain relief and exercise program preserves range of motion and strengthens muscles. If the rheumatoid arthritis becomes progressive and causes significant joint destruction, orthopedic surgeons are now able to replace many damaged joints.

The course of rheumatoid arthritis is unpredictable. Some patients have short-lived, acute attacks and then get better. Others suffer a chronic, progressive disease leading to joint damage and destruction. Many patients experience rheumatoid arthritis as a series of many episodes of marked inflammation and pain alternating with periods of mobility and relative freedom from pain. Historically, rheumatoid arthritis patients have often been the target of those promising relief through fad cures. Because spontaneous remission may be part of the natural course of acute rheumatoid arthritis, some patients may attribute their improvement to treatments that actually have no value. If, for example, spontaneous remission follows a visit to a radioactive mine in Utah, a diet of peanut butter or mushrooms, wearing a copper bracelet, or doing any of numerous things advertised in the popular media for the treatment of rheumatoid arthritis, these patients may mistake their remission for a cure, crediting whatever "treatment" preceded it.

For this reason, medical specialists and the Food and Drug Administration insist that any arthritis treatment, like any other medical therapy, be subject to a double-blind scientific study, one in which neither the physicians nor the patients being treated know whether the patients are receiving the active ingredient being tested or a placebo (an inactive substance). If medical investigators show, on objective measurements (data that can be evaluated independently), that patients receiving the active ingredient do better than those taking a placebo, then that treatment can be said to be successful to some degree. Few drugs or devices have passed this rigid test for rheumatoid arthritis.

In some patients with Sjogren's syndrome secondary to rheumatoid arthritis, an improvement in the rheumatoid arthritis may be accompanied by an improvement in the symptoms of Sjogren's syndrome as well. This may be related to the halt of the progressive dryness in various areas of the body as a generalized autoimmune response to treatment. In other cases, rheumatoid arthritis may be kept under control but the symptoms of Sjogren's disease will progress and worsen.

## Systemic Lupus Erythematosus

Lupus has many manifestations associated with a variety of auto-antibodies (antibodies that attack the body's own tissues and organs as if they are foreign). Virtually any part of the body can be involved in lupus. The illness can vary from a very mild disease, in which the patient has nothing more than some fatigue and joint discomfort, to one involving almost every organ system. Lupus can lead to death. With early diagnosis and effective treatment, mortality has decreased markedly over the last 10 years. Although lupus is predominantly an illness of women of childbearing age, it can affect almost any age group and occurs in men as well.

Many lupus patients have joint pains, with or without swelling, but these rarely lead to the deformities seen in rheumatoid arthritis. Muscle pain and weakness are commonly seen. Lupus patients often have various skin rashes; the most characteristic one, a butterfly rash, appears as a redness over the bridge of the nose and cheeks. Hair loss is quite common in lupus patients.

Organ system involvement in lupus can be very serious. In some patients, the linings of the lungs and heart are involved, leading to pleurisy and pericarditis. If the lungs themselves are affected, the patient may suffer pneumonias and hemorrhage into the lungs. Heart problems include cardiac failure and abnormalities of the coronary arteries. Kidney inflammation and damage leads to diffuse swelling of the body and eventual kidney failure. If lupus attacks the nervous system, various neurological problems may follow, among them seizures, strokes, psychoses, and various psychiatric and psychological problems.

Treatment of lupus is very complex and depends on the clinical signs and symptoms of the disease. Patients with only a skin rash and joint pain may require nothing more than aspirin and rest. Those who have progressive illness, or severe or frequent flareups, may require steroids, antimalarial medicines, immunosuppressive agents, or other drugs, which may decrease inflammation and stop the progression of the illness. Some patients with life-threatening disease may require kidney dialysis or treatments to control heart failure or high blood pressure. In a few patients, surgical replacement of diseased joints may also be necessary.

Lupus patients often have secondary Sjogren's syndrome. They too experience characteristic symptoms of dry eyes and dry mouth. Other lupus patients, however, have no symptoms of dryness and are totally unaware of the presence of Sjogren's syndrome. Yet when special tests are undertaken, inflammation of these glands is frequently found.

## Scleroderma

The most characteristic feature of scleroderma is a thickening and tightening of the skin due to excessive amounts of collagen, a protein normally present in skin. In scleroderma, excessive accumulation of collagen occurs for unknown reasons. Changes in the blood vessels and subtle reactions of the immune system are among the theories currently being investigated.

Scleroderma can be a very serious, life-threatening disorder. Internal organs may be damaged by the abnormal collagen accumulation. The gastrointestinal, pulmonary, cardiac, and renal systems may all be involved. Damage to the esophagus may lead to swallowing difficulties; diarrhea or malabsorption if the small intestine is affected; or constipation if the large bowel is involved. When the lungs and/or heart are affected, the patient may experience shortness of breath or cough, as in any other cardiopulmonary disease. Scleroderma is most serious when the kidneys are affected. Rapidly progressive kidney failure and markedly high blood pressure may follow as well. The blood vessels may be inflamed, causing ulcers and gangrene of the extremities. As many as 95 percent of scleroderma patients have Raynaud's phenomenon (see the next section). They may also experience pain, swelling, stiffening, and tightness of the joints. Muscle involvement may result in significant weakness. As in most connective tissue diseases, the severity of scleroderma varies. Scleroderma may involve minimal thickening in only one portion of the skin of the entire body may become leatherlike and all organ systems are damaged.

There is no specific treatment for scleroderma. Recent evidence, however, indicates that *d*-penicillamine, effective in the treatment of rheumatoid arthritis, may retard the progression of the disease. Generally, treatment is supportive. Pain relievers and anti-inflammatory medicines are used to control joint pain and stiffness. Physiotherapy is very important to maintain range of motion and prevent further contractures (shortening, producing distortion or deformity). Salves and emollients are used to soften the skin. When kidney problems and high blood pressure complicate the disease, various antihypertensive medicines are quite useful.

Sjogren's syndrome may complicate scleroderma, as it does rheumatoid arthritis, lupus, and polymyositis/dermatomyositis. It may be obvious in scleroderma patients who have dry eyes or a dry mouth. In others, it is found only when specifically sought through some of the special tests for Sjogren's syndrome.

### Raynaud's Phenomenon

In Raynaud's, the blood vessels, primarily in the arms, hands, legs, and feet, constrict on exposure to cold, and occasionally to other stimuli such as trauma or repeated impact. Women experience this problem more often than men. In the majority of cases, Raynaud's phenomenon is not a serious medical problem, though it can be quite uncomfortable. Some patients experience pain, tingling, and numbness when an episode occurs, while others feel only mild discomfort. In extreme cases, blood flow is decreased to the extent that ulceration and tissue damage occur. Consequent cracking of the skin and the formation of nonhealing ulcers are serious problems.

The clinical description of Raynaud's phenomenon is as follows: The fingers first turn white as the arterial blood vessels and capillaries constrict and less blood flows into the fingers; then the venous blood pools in the tissues, turning the fingers blue. As the episode subsides, a rush of new blood flows back into the fingers, turning them red. Thus, the classic sequence in Raynaud's phenomenon is from white to blue to red. As with all other connective tissue disorders, every patient has a unique profile. A patient may experience only the whitening or the blue phase, though this condition is still referred to as Raynaud's phenomenon. When the condition occurs alone, it is called Raynaud's disease; when it is associated with other connective tissue diseases, it is called Raynaud's phenomenon.

The appearance of Raynaud's presents problems for the clinician. The symptoms may be the first manifestation of a connective tissue disease such as lupus or scleroderma, or they may be the start of Raynaud's disease. A examination of the nail beds through an ophthalmoscope or a biomicroscope to find an identifiable pattern in blood vessels is valuable.

Medications are available for the treatment of Raynaud's. The ones most commonly used are calcium channel blockers, nifedipine, isradipine, and diltiazem, as well as many others. These medicines work by dilating blood vessels. They are also used in the treatment of angina and high blood pressure. Some patients respond favorably to nitroglycerin (commonly known as a treatment for angina) rubbed onto the fingers. Alpha channel blockers are also often used, the most common being Prazosin. Reserpine has also been used as a treatment. Since these drugs are associated with potential side effects, their use should be monitored carefully by a physician. Prostaglandin derivatives are under investigation as a potential treatment. Preliminary studies seem to indicate that certain patients with severe Raynaud's phenomenon, particularly those with scleroderma, may benefit.

Unresponsive Raynaud's may require surgery involving the sympathetic nerves in the neck or the fingers. Indications for this surgery are infrequent, but the procedure is available for the most severe cases.

Raynaud's patients can take an active role to minimize the effects of their disease. They can avoid exposure to the cold and wear warm clothing, especially warm socks and gloves. Biofeedback, a form of psychological training, may be helpful. Elimination of nicotine, which constricts blood vessels, is essential. When cutting the nails of the fingers and toes, the patient should not cut the cuticles. When using abrasive cleansers or materials such as steel wool that may break the skin, rubber or latex gloves should be worn. Repetitive impact to the extremities, as in the use of hand-held power tools, should be avoided.

### Polymyositis/Dermatomyositis

Polymyositis is an acquired (not inherited) disease of the muscles. Patients experience severe weakness in the major voluntary muscles. When accompanied by a characteristic rash, the disease is called dermatomyositis. Patients often complain of fatigue, as well as joint and muscle pain. However, the major symptom is weakness of the proximal muscles in the shoulder and hip girdle. The patient may have difficulty getting up from a chair, walking, getting out of a bathtub, raising the arms to comb the hair, or performing simple tasks. When the disease is profound, the patient may have no muscle strength at all.

Polymyositis may extend to the muscles of respiration, causing breathing difficulties, and to the muscles that control swallowing. Patients may have other symptoms normally associated with other connective tissue diseases, including joint pain, joint swelling, and Raynaud's phenomenon. Because polymyositis/dermatomyositis may be associated with a malignancy somewhere in the body, examination for such a condition should be part of the medical workup. The diagnosis of polymyositis/dermatomyositis is usually based on the clinical picture plus abnormalities in certain blood tests that suggest that the muscles are inflamed. The diagnosis of the disease is confirmed by electromyographic (EMG) studies and biopsy of involved muscle, which reveals the characteristic inflammation. However, occasionally the diagnosis is made in the absence of a positive biopsy.

Polymyositis/dermatomyositis can be very well controlled with corticosteroids and immunosuppressive medicines. Generally, physicians prescribe cortisone derivatives first and immunosuppressive medicines only if steroids fail or the amount necessary to control the disease causes unsatisfactory side effects. However, because the indications for using immunosuppressive medicines are not uniform among specialists, the treatment of polymyositis/dermatomyositis is in flux. Many patients go into spontaneous remission. Subtle symptoms of Sjogren's syndrome may occur in patients with polymyositis. When Sjogren's syndrome accompanies polymyositis, it is treated the same way as primary Sjogren's syndrome.

### Mixed Connective Tissue Disease

In the last few years, it has been recognized that some patients who have a connective tissue disease do not fall exactly into the categories previously described. Some controversy exists among clinicians regarding the diagnosis of mixed connective tissue disease. Since patients may simultaneously manifest some of the features of one or more of the diseases discussed above, some physicians see these patients as having overlap syndromes. Other physicians group these patients with a diagnosis of mixed connective tissue disease. Still others believe that patients with mixed connective tissue disease will eventually develop either scleroderma, Sjogren's syndrome, polymyositis, or lupus.

Until we know the specific causes of the connective tissue diseases, further research will be necessary to learn whether mixed connective tissue disease is a different entity or one of the other connective tissue diseases. One clinical finding has provided a clue: In addition to displaying a mixture of features normally associated with polymyositis, scleroderma, and lupus, mixed connective tissue disease patients have an antibody to an extractable nuclear antigen in their blood. This antigen, more specifically known as RNP or Ribonucleo-Protein, is thought to be characteristic of mixed connective tissue disease.

The treatment of mixed connective tissue disease depends principally on the symptoms. Patients with symptoms of polymyositis may respond to corticosteroids. If the principal manifestations are skin tightening or hardening, corticosteroids may be less effective.

### Vasculitis

In patients with primary Sjogren's syndrome, blood vessels can be affected in two ways. There may be either an inflammatory process (a collection of white blood cells inside and outside of the vessel wall leading to eventual destruction), called vasculitis, or/and other mechanisms that lead to conditions such as Raynaud's phenomenon and purpura.

### What Are the Factors?

Two biological processes are operating in the development of the vessel wall injury. First, immune complexes (clusters of antigens and their antibodies) are deposited on the vessel wall. These deposits successively activate a series of immunologically important blood proteins, called complement components, and induce inflammation and tissue destruction. Second, activated leukocytes (the white cells of the body's defense system) destroy the vessel wall.

During the inflammatory and subsequent healing process, narrowing and closing of the inside of the blood vessel result in ischemia (decreased blood supply) to the organs and tissues whose vessels are affected by the vasculitis. This is shown by the impaired function of these particular organs. The injury can lead to necrosis (tissue death).

### Which Sjogren's Syndrome Patients Develop Vasculitis?

The clinical experience of physicians treating Sjogren's syndrome patients suggests that vasculitis usually occurs several years after the diagnosis of primary Sjogren's syndrome has been established. Furthermore, primary Sjogren's syndrome patients affected by vasculitis are mainly those with more widespread extraglandular (outside the gland) disease. As a rule, vasculitis complicates Sjogren's syndrome that is not confined to the exocrine glands, that is, Sjogren's syndrome that is not limited to such manifestations as dry eyes and dry mouth. Vasculitis usually occurs in patients with Raynaud's phenomenon; enlarged lymph nodes, liver, and spleen; and kidney and lung involvement. In addition, serum cryoglobulins (specific protein complexes circulating in the blood that are deposited during cold exposure) are commonly detected.

### What Blood Vessels Are Involved and What Is the Clinical Picture of Sjogren's Syndrome Vasculitis?

The types of vessels affected by vasculitis in Sjogren's syndrome patients include (1) small vessels (arterioles, capillaries, and venules), which represent the minute terminal branches of arteries and veins, and (2) medium-sized arteries, for example, those that supply the bowel. Skin is the most commonly affected organ. Inflammation and destruction of capillaries and venules, with subsequent blood leakage, are responsible for the appearance of the skin. The Sjogren's syndrome patient with skin vasculitis usually has clusters of red/purple spots known as purpura.

The next most common symptom of vasculitis in Sjogren's syndrome patients is urticaria (hives), which may or may not contain petechiae (tiny red spots) and usually do not itch. Other, less commonly observed skin lesions include erythema multiforme (larger red spots with a pale center) and skin ulcers in the lower legs.

If the arteries supplying the fingers and toes are affected, a violet discoloration appears in these areas. It can progress to gangrene (tissue death) of the terminal part of a finger or toe.

Vasculitis of the small blood vessels supplying the nerves results in peripheral neuropathy, marked by numbness, tingling, pain, loss of sensation, and weakness in both hands and feet symmetrically in a so-called glove-and-stocking distribution. Sometimes a more serious problem occurs, called mononeuritis multiplex, meaning paralysis of one or more major nerve branches. This results in foot or hand paralysis. Myositis (muscle inflammation), usually mild, which manifests as diffuse muscle pains, is rather uncommon in Sjogren's syndrome but may be caused by a mild vasculitis involving the blood vessels of the muscles.

Very rarely, a vasculitis of medium-sized arteries may produce serious problems in Sjogren's syndrome patients. When the arteries supplying such organs as the small or large bowel or gallbladder are closed, the subsequent decrease in the blood supply to these organs can lead to necrosis and perforation, resulting in peritonitis (inflammation of the abdominal cavity). This can be fatal if not treated promptly with surgery.

Involvement of the small and medium-sized arteries supplying the kidneys leads to glomerular inflammation, producing a condition called glomerulonephritis. This is characterized clinically by peripheral edema (swelling), high blood pressure, and abnormal urine.

## How Do Physicians Diagnose Vasculitis in Sjogren's Syndrome Patients?

The first clue to the presence of vasculitis in Sjogren's syndrome patients is the symptoms that prompted the patient to seek medical attention.

Angiography (x-rays taken after a radiopaque dye is injected into the artery) may play a role in the diagnostic workup of Sjogren's syndrome patients with vasculitis, as it does in polyarteritis nodosa patients, in whom it may reveal characteristic microaneurysms (small sacs) of the arterial wall.

The diagnosis of vasculitis in Sjogren's syndrome patients is confirmed by biopsy. If the skin is involved, biopsy of an area with lesions will disclose the characteristic picture of small vessel vasculitis. In cases of neuropathy, biopsy of a sural nerve (a small nerve branch in the calf of the leg) may confirm the diagnosis. Muscle biopsy may reveal a similar inflammation in the vessels supplying the muscle with blood.

Additional laboratory abnormalities observed in Sjogren's syndrome patients with vasculitis include a high erythrocyte (red blood cell) sedimentation rate, anemia, cryoglobulins in the serum, low complement

---

TABLE 6   PREVALENCE OF LABORATORY
ABNORMALITIES IN NINE PRIMARY
SJOGREN'S SYNDROME PATIENTS
WITH VASCULITIS

| Laboratory Abnormality | Number of Patients |
| --- | --- |
| Increased gamma globulins | 7 |
| Positive RF | 9 |
| Positive ANA | 9 |
| Cryoglobulins in serum | 9 |
| Low serum complement | 7 |

---

levels (indicating their consumption in the inflammatory process), and high levels of specific autoantibodies (antibodies against self) such as rheumatoid factor (RF) and antinuclear antibodies (ANA). Figures on these laboratory abnormalities, obtained from a recent study, appear in Table 6.

### How Do Physicians Treat Vasculitis in Sjogren's Syndrome Patients and What Is the Prognosis?

If skin involvement is the only manifestation of vasculitis in a Sjogren's syndrome patient, this condition is benign and specific measures are not necessary. The physician usually recommends only that the patient keep the legs elevated to avoid the aggravating effect of gravity on the development of petechiae (red spots).

The term benign could, with some reservations, be applied to most other manifestations of vasculitis in Sjogren's syndrome patients. This is because Sjogren's syndrome patients with vasculitis usually respond well to appropriate treatment, better than do patients with other forms of idiopathic (of unknown cause) vasculitis. In Sjogren's syndrome patients whose muscles, kidneys, or nerves are affected by vasculitis, drugs such as corticosteroids and cyclophosphamide (a medication that suppresses the immune response, given either by mouth or by intermittent intravenous injections) are necessary and the results are beneficial.

Sometimes, especially when the serious manifestations noted above are related to cryoglobulins circulating in the blood, the physician will recommend plasmapheresis, a technique in which the patient's blood is removed by a machine similar to a dialysis machine and cleansed of circulating immune complexes and cryoglobulins.

Finally, in a patient in whom vasculitis causes perforation of an abdominal organ and peritonitis, the prognosis depends on the promptness of surgical intervention.

## Why Sjogren's Syndrome Is Believed to Be an Autoimmune Disease

When secondary Sjogren's syndrome is associated with connective tissue diseases such as rheumatoid arthritis and systemic lupus erythematosus, an autoimmune process is presumed to underlie the syndrome. However, physicians often see primary Sjogren's syndrome patients who have various features of autoimmunity, including inflammation of the joints, kidneys, liver, and gastrointestinal tract, who do not fall into any of the strict categories of connective tissue diseases described above. For example, patients who receive a graft from another individual may develop graft-versus-host disease, in which the host seems to reject the graft by means of an immunological reaction. These patients often have a disorder that is nearly identical to Sjogren's syndrome as well. This suggests that primary Sjogren's syndrome is also a result of autoimmunity.

## Breast Implants and Rheumatic Diseases
### The Relationship Between Silicone Implants and Connective Tissue Diseases

It has been estimated that over 2 million women have had silicone breast implants. Though some are done for reconstruction after breast surgery, the majority are done for cosmetic purposes. The use of silicone breast implants and silicone capsules has been extremely popular. Prior to the use of implants, attempts at breast augmentation using paraffin or free silicone injections led to unacceptable cosmetic results and many complications. The use of free silicone injections to augment and repair tissues was never approved by the Food and Drug Administration.

Over the years, a number of sporadic reports focused on the possible association between silicone implants and various autoimmune connective tissue diseases. In 1988, Dr. Spiera published an article about a series of patients with scleroderma who had breast implants. He demonstrated that 5 of 106 consecutive patients with scleroderma had breast implants compared to only 1 of 286 patients with rheumatoid arthritis, suggesting that breast implants might be a risk factor for the development of scleroderma. Since that time, there has been great interest among physicians, the press, and the legal community about this possible association.

In addition to scleroderma, the diseases potentially associated with silicone implants are rheumatoid arthritis, lupus, Sjogren's syndrome, polymyositis/dermatomyositis, and various nonspecific rheumatic diseases. There is clear evidence that even in patients with no rupture of the capsule, silicone may be found outside the implant. It is not clear whether this causes disease.

Several studies seem to suggest that there is no excessive number of rheumatic or connective tissue diseases in patients with implants. On the other hand, many women with nonspecific musculoskeletal findings with rheumatic and other symptoms feel that the breast implants somehow adversely affected their health. This subject is being studied in academic institutions and by breast implant manufacturers. At present, it is the cause of a great deal of litigation. However, there is no convincing evidence that silicone implants have a statistically significant association with Sjogren's syndrome or other connective tissue diseases.

Unfortunately, there are no hard data that show a clear association between silicone implants and various connective tissues diseases. It should be noted that silicone implants include chin and toe implants as well as breast implants, though breast implants are by far the most common. The evidence to date seems to suggest that if any disease is associated with the implants, the most likely candidate is scleroderma.

The rheumatic diseases occur commonly in the general population. It is estimated that 1 percent of women have rheumatoid arthritis, 500 per million have systemic lupus, and 50 per million have scleroderma. Any assessment of the association between implants and rheumatic diseases must consider the background frequency of these diseases. To date, it does not seem that more patients with silicone implants have developed rheumatoid arthritis or clearly defined lupus than would be expected on the basis of chance alone. For scleroderma, on the other hand, more patients have already been described in the medical literature than would be expected on the basis of chance alone. A more definitive answer will have to await the results of ongoing research.

Should a woman who develops a connective tissue disease have the implant removed? Once again, there are not enough definitive studies on which to base unequivocal advice. We suggest the following approach. If a patient with a silicone implant has a life- or organ-threatening disease, we recommend implant removal to see if it has a beneficial effect. If under other circumstances we would use an aggressive treatment that itself would have major side effects, we would recommend the removal of the implant first. Otherwise, if the patient is satisfied with the cosmetic results of the implant, we may not have enough evidence to reach any clear conclusion. In a questionnaire sent to 30 patients seen by Dr. Spiera, a clear majority said that having their implants removed had no effect on their connective tissue disorder.

In the 16 patients on whom Dr. Spiera has the most information, that is, those patients with scleroderma, 8 had the implants removed. Two seemed to have mild improvement in their disease. In two others, removal made no difference at all, and four clearly had progression of their disease after removal. Again, it is not clear in these cases that the implant was the cause of the scleroderma. Any woman with a breast implant and a connective tissue disease must contact her physician to decide on the best course of action on an individual basis. Hopefully, ongoing research will allow a more definitive answer concerning both the relationship of the implants to connective tissue diseases and how such diseases should be handled in patients who have had implants.

# 9 Pulmonary Conditions

THE UPPER AIRWAY (mouth, throat, and nose), the lower airway (trachea or windpipe), and its branches (the bronchi), and the lungs themselves may be involved in Sjogren's syndrome. Mucous gland dysfunction is the hallmark of Sjogren's syndrome, and the internal linings of the upper and lower airways and the lungs contain mucous glands. Microscopically, the glands are found to be flooded with lymphocytes (white blood cells), which are thought to cause the dysfunction.

The precise incidence of pulmonary (pertaining to the air passages and lungs) involvement in Sjogren's syndrome is uncertain. Estimates range from 1 percent to 60 percent. Because pulmonary disorders are commonly seen in association with other autoimmune diseases (in which the immune system mistakenly attacks the body's own tissues or organs), such as rheumatoid arthritis, systemic lupus erythematosus, and scleroderma, at times it may be difficult to separate the forms of pulmonary involvement commonly seen in these diseases from those that are peculiar to Sjogren's syndrome.

## Aspiration Pneumonia

Xerostomia (dry mouth) causes pulmonary problems in two ways. First, a dry mouth not only makes swallowing difficult, it makes it impossible to soften food well enough to pass it to the back of the throat and into the esophagus. Occasionally, food or liquid goes the wrong way and is aspirated into the lungs. The patient coughs to clear the lungs of the foreign material. Sometimes the food particles remain in the lungs and cause a pneumonia called aspiration pneumonia. The cardinal symp-

---

**TABLE 7   PULMONARY MANIFESTATIONS OF SJOGREN'S SYNDROME**

---

*Upper Respiratory Tract*

Atrophic rhinitis (nasal dryness)
Xerostomia (dry mouth)


*Lower Respiratory Tract*

Tracheobronchitis (dryness of the tracheobronchial tree, made up of the trachea and its
  branches, the bronchi)
Recurrent infections
Bronchitis (infection of the bronchial tubes, leading to fever, cough, and sputum)
Bronchiectasis (weakening of the bronchial tubes, leading to chronic cough and sputum
  production)
Acute pneumonia/lung abscess (serious lung infection with resultant cavity)
Bronchiolitis* (inflammation and scar tissue in the substance of the lung)
Atelectasis* (partial collapse of a lung segment, often with mucous plugging)
Interstitial pneumonia, chronic* (inflammation and scar tissue in the substance of the
  lung)
Pleurisy* (inflammation of the pleura, the lungs' lining)
Pulmonary hypertension and vasculitis* (high pressure in the lungs' blood vessels)
Amyloidosis (formation of a starch-like substance in the lungs)
Diaphragmatic dysfunction* (disorder of the muscle separating the abdomen and the
  heart and lung cavity)
Pseudolymphoma (an abnormal accumulation of lymphocytes, either in the interstitium
  of the lung or in lymph glands in the center of the chest)
Lymphoma (cancer of the lymph glands) involving the lungs
Disordered breathing during sleep (sleep apnea, fatigue)

---

* Disorders found in other collagen vascular diseases.

---

toms of this pneumonia are cough, sputum, fever, and, in severe cases, shortness of breath. Confirmed by a standard chest x-ray, aspiration pneumonia is treated with antibiotics and usually requires hospitalization.

## Anaerobic Pneumonia and Lung Abscess

Because a dry mouth also leads to dental caries (cavities) and gingival (gum) infection, bacteria from the tooth or gum infection may be passed into the lung, either during sleep or because of ineffective swallowing. This leads to a type of pneumonia often caused by anaerobic bacteria (bacteria that grow best without oxygen). If not properly treated, anaerobic pneumonia commonly leads to a lung abscess.

The patient may have anaerobic pneumonia and lung abscess for weeks or months before it becomes apparent. The symptoms are weight loss, fever, and foul-smelling or foul-tasting sputum. Anaerobic pneumonia, diagnosed on the basis of the patient's history and a chest x-ray, requires several weeks of treatment with antibiotics such as penicillin or clindamycin. Since Sjogren's syndrome patients have a higher than normal incidence of side effects from antibiotics, particularly certain types of penicillin, drug therapy must be individualized.

## Esophageal Problems

Regurgitation of food or drink may be caused by abnormalities of the esophagus in Sjogren's syndrome patients. These problems, including esophageal hypomotility (loss of the usual muscular contractions in the esophagus that propel food from the mouth to the stomach), achalasia (muscular spasm in the lower portion of the esophagus), and webs (bands of tissue blocking the opening of the esophagus) are thoroughly discussed in Chapter 10. Medication directed at the underlying problem or surgical intervention may be required.

## Laryngotracheobronchitis

Laryngotracheobronchitis (chronic inflammation of the voice box, windpipe, and bronchial tubes, punctuated by acute infectious episodes) is caused by mucous gland dysfunction in Sjogren's syndrome patients. When mucous production decreases, both in quality and in quantity, the Sjogren's syndrome patient is unable to clear foreign matter that has been inhaled into the respiratory tract.

Cough, the main symptom of laryngotracheobronchitis, can be debilitating. Ineffective coughing due to fatigue or malnutrition results in mucus becoming inspissated (thickened and stuck in the bronchi), leading to atelectasis (collapse of a segment of lung due to the lack of ventilation to that area). Eventually, pneumonia may result.

## Tracheobronchitis

Mild tracheobronchitis (inflammation of the windpipe and bronchial tubes) is quite common in Sjogren's syndrome patients. Some studies have suggested an incidence of up to 50 percent. Symptoms include chest burning, pain associated with breathing, shortness of breath, wheezing, and hoarseness of the voice.

In contrast to its usefulness in diagnosing pneumonia, a standard chest x-ray is usually normal and not helpful in diagnosing tracheo-bronchitis. Results of pulmonary function (breathing) tests are more sensitive in supporting the patient's history. Although there are many types of breathing tests, the diagnosis of tracheobronchitis may be confirmed by simple spirometry. In this test, which may be performed in the doctor's office, the patient is asked to take a deep breath and then exhale into a tube as rapidly as possible, repeating this procedure several times. In tracheobronchitis the vital capacity (total amount of air exhaled) may be normal, but the rate at which the air is exhaled is slow. This indicates an obstructive ventilatory impairment or blockage of air flow. If the physician suspects that this condition is present, even though the routine tests have been normal, a special type of pulmonary function test, the methacholine challenge test, may be required.

### Treatments for Relief of Tracheobronchitis

Humidifying mists from properly cleaned room humidifiers or medically prescribed nebulizers may be helpful. Nebulizers break up water droplets into fine microscopic particles, which are freely suspended in the air and thus capable of reaching the smallest bronchioles.

If the patient is wheezing or if a blockage to air flow is found on pulmonary function tests, then bronchodilator medications may be prescribed. These medications, which come in tablet, capsule, or aerosol mist form, relax the smooth muscle surrounding the bronchial tubes, partially relieving the blockage.

Bronchodilators must be used with caution, especially in persons with cardiovascular diseases. Occasional side effects include palpitations (rapid or irregular heartbeat), tremor, insomnia, anxiety, and gastrointestinal upsets such as nausea, vomiting, and diarrhea.

Numerous types of methyl xanthines may be given orally or intravenously. Methyl xanthines that may be used in tracheobronchitis are primarily theophylline and aminophylline (e.g., Theodur, Theolair, Slo-Bid, and Uniphyl). If bronchodilators and methyl xanthines are not helpful, the physician may try corticosteroids such as prednisone, Medrol, or cortisone. Inhaled corticosteroids, which may be of use in tracheobronchitis, include Vanceril (Beclomethasone), Aerobid, (Flusinolide), Azmacort (Triamcinolone), Flouent (Fluticosone), and Pulmicort (Bidesonide). Corticosteroids have both anti-inflammatory and bronchodilator properties. In many cases, they destroy the abnormal accumulation of lymphocytes in the mucous glands of the tracheobronchial tree and are successful in treating tracheobronchitis in Sjogren's syndrome patients. Corticosteroids taken orally may have serious side effects if taken at high doses or for prolonged periods. They must be taken under close medical supervision for only severe manifestations of Sjogren's syndrome, whether for pulmonary symptoms or for symptoms in other parts of the body.

## Bronchiolitis

Bronchiolitis (inflammation of bronchial tube branches less than 2 mm in diameter) has been recognized only recently as a problem for Sjogren's syndrome patients. As a result of accumulated lymphocytes in the mucous glands, bronchioles may become permanently obstructed by mucus or scar tissue.

Once believed to be rare, bronchiolitis is now thought to be fairly common in Sjogren's syndrome. In one study, the disorder was found in 6 of 13 Sjogren's syndrome patients but was serious in only 2. Although the prognosis for patients with broncholitis is usually poor, it may improve if the disease is recognized and treated earlier.

As in tracheobronchitis, pulmonary function tests, chiefly spirometry, are most helpful in making the diagnosis. Chest x-rays are less useful.

## Interstitial Pneumonia

As the bronchi branch successively into bronchioles, they end in microscopic air sacs called alveoli. The millions of alveoli in the lungs are embedded in supporting tissue known as the interstitium. Within the interstitium are capillaries (tiny blood vessels) that take oxygen from and give carbon dioxide to the alveoli.

In interstitial pneumonia, an abnormal accumulation of lymphocytes (white blood cells) and scar tissue in the supporting tissue around the alveoli forms a barrier to the speedy exchange of oxygen and carbon dioxide between the alveoli and the capillaries. As the blood oxygen content drops, organs throughout the body may malfunction. The patient complains of shortness of breath on exertion. As the lungs become abnormally stiff, the patient develops a rapid, shallow breathing pattern. Although cough is a common symptom, sputum production is less likely. The chest x-ray and pulmonary function tests are abnormal. Pulmonary function tests measure a reduced volume of air in the lungs, while the rate of air entry and exit is normal or supernormal.

An additional pulmonary function test for early indications of interstitial pneumonia in Sjogren's syndrome is the diffusing capacity test, which measures the rate of gas transfer from the air sacs to the lungs' blood vessels. This test may be done in a pulmonary specialist's office or in a hospital pulmonary function laboratory.

The severity of interstitial pneumonia may vary from no symptoms to a disabling shortness of breath at rest. Lymphocytic interstitial pneumonia, a form of interstitial pneumonia most often seen in Sjogren's syndrome, is usually treated with corticosteroids. It does not cause long-term disability. If not treated early, interstitial pneumonia may progress to an end stage and may be untreatable.

### Interstitial Pneumonitis

The distinction between interstitial pneumonia and interstitial pneumonitis (inflammation of the supporting tissue around the alveoli of the lungs) is subtle. A recent study suggests that many Sjogren's syndrome patients may have interstitial pneumonitis long before symptoms appear or before the chest x-ray and pulmonary function tests become abnormal.

Two relatively new techniques, the gallium scan and bronchoscopy with bronchoalveolar lavage, are used to detect inflammation in the lung. In gallium scanning, the patient is given an injection of gallium, a radioisotope, which is taken up in areas of inflammation throughout the body. After 48 to 72 hours, lung inflammation will show up on a scan of the lungs. Bronchoalveolar lavage (flushing the lungs with saline) is performed at the time of bronchoscopy (putting a tube into the lungs).

Interstitial pneumonitis is treated with corticosteroids when there is evidence of a clear-cut deterioration in lung function. The Sjogren's syndrome patient is given a trial of corticosteroids and reassessed at the end of 4 to 6 weeks. If the patient has had a good response, the dose is slowly lowered and the patient closely monitored for possible relapse. If the patient has not improved after 6 weeks, corticosteroids should be discontinued because the risk of harmful side effects begins to outweigh the possible benefits.

### Distinguishing Interstitial Pneumonitis from Other Conditions

Interstitial pneumonitis in Sjogren's syndrome patients needs to be differentiated from infection, pseudolymphoma (an abnormally high accumulation of lymphocytes in the lungs or lymph glands of the chest), lymphona (cancer of the lymph glands), and other conditions. Therefore, a lung biopsy is often needed.

A lung biopsy is performed either through a standard thoracotomy chest incision or by video assisted thoracoscopy (open lung biopsy) under general anesthesia or through a flexible bronchoscope, a narrow tube that enables the physician to see into the bronchial tubes. While the patient is awake under local anesthesia, the bronchoscope is passed through the nose. Biopsies taken via bronchoscopy are satisfactory for excluding infection but may not provide a large or representative enough sample to distinguish between inflammatory and tumorous conditions. In these cases, an open lung biopsy may be advisable.

### Pleurisy

Pleurisy (inflammation of the lining around the lungs) usually causes chest or shoulder pain on breathing. Pleural effusion (fluid accumulation in the pleural space) may lead to shortness of breath. Pleurisy is treated with corticosteroids, as well as nonsteroidal anti-inflammatory drugs. In some cases, drainage of fluid may be necessary.

### Pulmonary Hypertension

Pulmonary hypertension is an abnormally high pressure in the pulmonary arteries, the blood vessels carrying blood from the heart to the lungs. Drugs designed to dilate pulmonary arteries are used, such as nitroglycerine, nifedipine (Procardia), prostacyclin, and hydralazine.

### Pulmonary Pseudolymphoma

Pulmonary pseudolymphoma is an abnormal accumulation of lymphocytes, either in the interstitium (supporting tissue lining the air sacs or alveoli) of the lung or in the lymph glands in the mediastinum, the center of the chest. Microscopically and on x-ray, pseudolymphoma may resemble lymphoma, a malignant tumor of the lymph glands.

Pseudolymphoma may be asymptomatic, appearing only on a routine x-ray. Alternatively, by putting pressure on nearby lung structures, it may cause chest pain, cough, wheezing, or shortness of breath. To make the diagnosis, a lymph node or lung biopsy is necessary. The slides taken from the biopsied tissue should be reviewed by a pathologist experienced in differentiating benign pseudolymphoma from malignant lymphoma. Newer pathological staining techniques of lymphoid tissue have greatly enhanced the ability to differentiate between benign and malignant disorders. This distinction is often difficult, and experts may disagree.

The prognosis for pseudolymphoma is good. It may improve spontaneously or may need treatment with corticosteroids. In a very few cases, pseudolymphoma develops into a malignant lymphoma.

## Lymphoma

Lymphoma (cancer of the lymph glands; see Chapter 13) develops in a small percentage (less than 5 percent) of Sjogren's syndrome patients, more commonly in those who do not have an associated collagen vascular disorder. It may affect any organ in the body, commonly causing fever, weight loss, anemia, night sweats, and itching of the skin. Pulmonary symptoms are similar to those of pseudolymphoma.

A lymph node biopsy must be performed to make the diagnosis. Treatment may include radiation therapy and/or chemotherapy, with or without corticosteroids. The prognosis is variable.

David Eskreis, MD

# 10 Disorders of the Gastrointestinal System

SJOGREN'S SYNDROME is an increasingly recognized rheumatological disorder that affects primarily middle-aged and elderly women. The early description of this disorder by Henrik Sjogren included the symptoms of dry eyes (xerophthalmia) and dry mouth (xerostomia). These symptoms remain the cornerstone of diagnosis. Gastrointestinal symptoms are common in patients with Sjogren's syndrome. The esophagus, stomach, and liver are the organs most frequently involved.

## Esophagus

The esophagus is a hollow muscular tube that squeezes food from the mouth to the stomach. When it functions abnormally, painful swallowing is a result, symptoms of food sticking and chest pressure are frequent complaints and are not due to dryness of the mouth alone.

Heartburn (pyrosis) is common and is due to laxity of the muscle separating the esophagus and stomach. This leads to acid regurgitation compounded by the loss of the acid-neutralizing properties of saliva. This may lead to esophageal inflammation, with resultant bleeding, scarring, or malignancy.

Less common causes of swallowing difficulties in Sjogren's syndrome are cricoid webs and achalasia. A cricoid web is a band-like narrowing of tissue occurring high in the esophagus. It may be asymptomatic or may cause coughing, choking, and neck pain. These webs are associated with iron deficiency anemia, ulcerative colitis, and various thyroid disorders. The diagnosis is made by a physician using x-ray or examination with a fiberoptic instrument.

Achalasia is a disorder caused by weak peristaltic contractions of the esophagus and impaired lower esophageal sphincter muscle relaxation. Symptoms include difficulty swallowing, chest pressure, nausea, vomiting, and malodorous breath. Nighttime heartburn and choking on regurgitated esophageal contents may lead to recurrent pneumonia and asthma.

### Stomach

The stomach is primarily a storage organ delivering food at a controlled rate into the small intestine for digestion. The stomach lining contains specialized cells that form acid, mucus, and a protein called intrinsic factor, the last required for vitamin $B_{12}$ absorption. The stomach lining may become inflamed, a condition known as gastritis. When the gastritis leads to loss of the specialized lining cells, the lining becomes flat or atrophic. It is estimated that 40 percent of patients over the age of 45 have atrophic gastritis, but almost 80 percent of Sjogren's syndrome patients of the same age have this disorder.

Patients with atrophic gastritis complain of abdominal pain, nausea, bloating, and loss of appetite. In contrast to patients with the more common peptic inflammation of the stomach, these patients do not respond to acid reduction. The armamentarium of liquid antacids, H2 blockers, and proton pump inhibitors generally provides little symptomatic relief.

### Small Intestine

The small intestine is infrequently involved in Sjogren's syndrome. A few cases of celiac sprue, a disease of malabsorption of grains, have been associated with this condition. Only a single case of Crohn's disease has been reported.

### Pancreas

The pancreas is important in controlling blood sugar and releasing digestive enzymes. Pancreatic disease therefore may occur with irregularities of sugar balance, diarrhea, and/or weight loss. The diarrhea and weight loss are a result of impaired food absorption related to decreased release of digestive enzymes.

Pancreatitis is an inflammatory disease of the pancreas resulting in abdominal pain and elevated blood levels of the pancreatic enzyme amylase. The most common causes of pancreatitis are alcohol abuse and gallstones, but pancreatitis in Sjogren's syndrome is due to an unknown cause. Rare cases of chronic pancreatitis have been reported in Sjogren's syndrome patients. Four cases of chronic pancreatitis, primary sclerosing cholangitis, and Sjogren's syndrome have been reported.

Microscopically, the salivary glands and pancreas have a similar structure. The salivary glands also store amylase, releasing it into the salivary fluid to aid in digestion of sugars. Most Sjogren's syndrome patients have salivary gland inflammation, and thus the blood amylase level is commonly elevated. Differentiating between $p$-amylase (pancreatic) and $s$-amylase (salivary) can be done only in specialized laboratories.

If a person with Sjogren's syndrome goes to an emergency room with abdominal pain and elevated amylase, the diagnosis of pancreatitis will be suspected and may be correct. However, the elevated amylase may be normal for this person. It may be of salivary and not pancreatic origin. Therefore, patients must be knowledgeable about their disease and let the physician caring for them know that they have Sjogren's syndrome. This may change the direction of the patients' medical evaluation and treatment.

## Liver

Many liver disorders are initiated or perpetuated by abnormalities of the immune system. Therefore, it is not surprising that they are associated with Sjogren's syndrome, which is an autoimmune disease. In one study of liver abnormalities in patients with Sjogren's syndrome, elevated liver function tests were found in 25 percent of patients and liver enlargement in 33 percent. The strongest association between Sjogren's syndrome and liver disease exists in patients with primary biliary cirrhosis (PBC). Symptoms of Sjogren's syndrome are reported in about 70 percent of patients with PBC. This is a liver disorder of middle-aged women with fatigue and itching. It leads to progressive liver damage and cirrhosis over two to three decades.

Hepatitis caused by viruses may lead to chronic inflammation of the liver and eventual cirrhosis. Hepatitis B and hepatitis C (the latter previously called non-A/non-B hepatitis) are associated with Sjogren's syndrome symptoms in up to 40 percent of patients. Dry eyes seem to be more common than dry mouth. Symptoms severe enough to warrant treatment occur in 10 percent of patients with chronic hepatitis.

Autoimmune hepatitis, another disease of middle-aged women characterized by an elevated level of antinuclear antibodies (which attack the body's tissues and organs as if they are foreign) and arthritis, is also associated with Sjogren's syndrome. This form of hepatitis is treatable with corticosteroids and may also progress to cirrhosis if untreated.

In summary, the manifestations of Sjogren's syndrome are multiple, and gastrointestinal involvement is common. The esophagus and stomach are the organs most often affected in the Sjogren's syndrome patient. Pancreatic disease can occur in Sjogren's syndrome, but elevation of amylase may be due to salivary inflammation and may be confused with pancreatitis. Patients with chronic liver disease, especially PBC, have a high incidence of symptoms related to Sjogren's syndrome.

Stuart S. Kassan, MD, FACP

Robert J. Kassan, MD

# 11 Kidney Involvement

LONG RECOGNIZED as a complex condition responsible for dryness of the eyes, nose, and mouth, Sjogren's syndrome also involves extraglandular (outside the glands) organs and systems. Not the least of these is the renal or kidney system.

Kidney conditions can occur in both primary Sjogren's syndrome, in which the sicca (dryness) complex is not associated with an underlying disease, and secondary Sjogren's syndrome, in which the patient has an associated connective tissue disorder, particularly rheumatoid arthritis or systemic lupus erythematosus.

In either case, the basic problem is similar. Something has gone wrong with the immune system, the body's defense against disease. White blood cells, called lymphocytes, are overproduced and invade the body's tissues, interfering with normal functions such as the production of tears and saliva. The lymphocytes produce unusual proteins, called autoantibodies, which may also lead to organ malfunction.

A similar process occurs when the kidneys are affected in Sjógren's syndrome. Immune elements, including lymphocytes, antibodies, cryo-globulins (a form of protein in the blood), and an unusual macroglobulin (large protein) are deposited in the kidney tissues. In some instances, the exact location and extent of involvement can be determined by means of a kidney biopsy.

## Manifestations of Kidney Disease

Kidney diseases in Sjogren's syndrome are of several types, depending on which element of the renal system is involved. A thorough study, including a history of the patient, is important.

The most common kidney condition seen in Sjogren's syndrome patients is interstitial nephritis, which is inflammation in the kidney tissue surrounding the filtering elements. Because this causes difficulty in producing a concentrated urine, patients with interstitial nephritis urinate more frequently than normal and in larger quantities.

Sjogren's syndrome patients may have a condition known as renal tubular acidosis, in which they are unable to excrete highly acid urine. This may cause a severe depletion of potassium in the blood, resulting in an electrolyte imbalance, a condition in which the amounts of normal essential blood chemicals such as sodium, chloride, carbon dioxide, calcium, phosphorus, and urea nitrogen, as well as potassium, are changed. These alterations can result in the impairment of important physiological functions, including heart action, muscle contraction, and nerve conduction. Also important is the possible lowering of the normal pH value in the blood, which has little room for variation. The lowering of the pH value, indicating an acidity reaction, will result in an acidosis.

In many instances, renal tubular acidosis has no obvious clinical symptoms, so the condition is unrecognized. At other times, kidney symptoms may appear before the sicca symptoms. Other findings include calcification of the kidney, kidney stones, and a lower than normal urinary citrate concentration.

Occasionally, a Sjogren's syndrome patient will have a true glomerulonephritis, an inflammation of the glomerulus, or filtering element of the kidney. This occurs because the immune complex has been deposited only in this part of the kidney. One group of investigators noted an associated purpura (areas of bleeding in the skin), hematuria (blood in the urine), proteinuria (albumin in the urine), and marked hypertension. These patients also had high levels of rheumatoid factor (a titer greater than 1:640) and moderate levels of antinuclear antibodies (a titer greater than 1:160).

Other areas of the urinary tract may also be affected in Sjogren's syndrome patients. Interstitial cystitis, a chronic nonbacterial inflammation of the bladder, occurs rarely in these patients. It may be associated with painful urination. Pseudolymphoma (a rare tumor seen in Sjogren's syndrome patients; see Chapter 13) may be found in the urinary tract, causing blockage in the flow of urine.

## Diagnostic Tests

Whenever a patient has a definite or suspected case of Sjogren's syndrome, the investigation of all systems, including the renal system, must be thorough because of the wide range of possible disorders. Some of these problems are latent, often causing no symptoms for long periods of time.

Whenever the physician suspects the possibility of Sjogren's syndrome, a complete study of the kidney must be conducted. This study should include measurements of electrolytes (blood sodium, potassium, chloride, and bicarbonate), as well as blood urea nitrogen and serum creatinine. In addition, the urine should be studied for albumin and a determination of the reaction (pH value). A 24-hour urine test for creatinine clearance should be completed.

If the patient has had kidney symptoms for a long time, a sonogram or an intravenous pyelogram (IVP), a kidney x-ray taken after an opaque dye has been injected into the bloodstream, may be required to determine the possible presence of calcium deposits.

In rare instances, when there is marked kidney impairment, a kidney biopsy may be necessary.

## Treatments

There is no specific treatment for kidney involvement in Sjogren's syndrome. In many instances, particularly in interstitial nephritis and renal tubular acidosis, the abnormalities are latent and require no treatment. However, regular follow-up is strongly suggested. With more overt manifestations of disease, specifically kidney stones, calcification of the kidney, and elevated urinary pH values, alkaline agents are used to prevent or reverse the potential development of metabolic acidosis (lowered pH values) and to prevent lowered potassium values.

In some cases, when progressive renal insufficiency develops and specifically when renal function worsens, a kidney biopsy may be done. Depending on the findings, corticosteroid (prednisone or methylprednisolone) therapy may be used. In more severe cases, immunosuppressive therapy (chemotherapy) may be needed (e.g., azathioprine, cyclophosphamide).

The most common adverse reactions to immunosuppressive therapy include mouth ulcers, leukopenia (lowered white blood cell count), nausea, and abdominal distress. In addition, there may be chills and fever, loss of hair, skin rashes, bone marrow depression, and kidney involvement, resulting in failing function. In view of the potentially serious and sometimes life-threatening reactions to immunosuppressive drugs, their use must be considered carefully.

## Conclusion

Kidney involvement in Sjogren's syndrome is not uncommon. However, the percentage of patients with overt clinical manifestations is small. Many cases can be determined only by specific tests. When there is evidence of progressive deterioration of kidney function, frequent observation is necessary and appropriate tests should be performed. Depending on the findings, aggressive therapy should be pursued in an attempt to control the progress of failing kidney function. Nothing takes the place of a periodic history, a physical exam, and frequent follow-up.

# 12 Nervous System Disorders

ALTHOUGH SJOGREN'S SYNDROME mainly affects the exocrine glands, in particular the glands producing tears and saliva, it has the potential to strike other organ systems. A frequent target of this extraglandular assault is the nervous system. Fortunately, nervous system disturbances occur in only a minority of patients with Sjogren's syndrome.

## Organization of the Nervous System

The nervous system is organized into pathways with cells and projections that transfer complex information about what we sense, where we move, and how we think and speak. The heart of this biological unit is the brain and spinal cord, or central nervous system. The brain supports our higher functions, including those of perception, spatial relationships, language, purposeful movement, sensation, memory, emotion, hearing, and sight. The spinal cord serves as a relay station to convey sensory and motor (movement) information between the brain and the rest of the body. The spinal cord also contains the circuitry for several reflex responses. The cranial nerves, spinal nerves, and peripheral nerves comprise the peripheral nervous system. The cranial nerves supply sensation and motor function to the eyes, ears, face, jaw, throat, and tongue. The spinal nerves originate from the spinal cord and give rise to the peripheral nerves that supply sharply defined areas of motor and sensory function. The peripheral nerves contain axons, or nerve fibers, that conduct electrical impulses to specialized receptors in the skin and muscles. The receptors in the skin are able to detect changes in pressure, pain, and temperature. This information is then transmitted through the peripheral nerves, up the spinal cord, and finally to the brain, where it is integrated and processed to create our sensory perceptions. Peripheral nerve fibers of another type terminate on receptors in muscle, carrying signals from the brain and spinal cord that trigger muscle contraction and produce movement.

## Carpal Tunnel Syndrome

The division of the nervous system most frequently involved in Sjogren's syndrome is the peripheral nervous system. A peripheral nerve disorder that occurs commonly in Sjogren's syndrome is carpal tunnel syndrome. This condition is termed an entrapment neuropathy because abnormal tissue (e.g., swollen joint tissue) accumulates in the carpal tunnel and compresses, or traps, the median nerve. Entrapment of the median nerve produces pain, numbness, and tingling of the thumb, index, and middle fingers and, in more advanced cases, muscle weakness. Sleep is frequently disturbed due to these abnormal sensations.

A careful medical history and a physical examination will usually reveal the telltale clues of carpal tunnel syndrome. If necessary, the diagnosis may be confirmed by performing nerve conduction velocity studies, which in most cases will demonstrate the slowing of electrical impulses in this part of the median nerve. The treatment of carpal tunnel syndrome may start with the use of a lightweight canvas wrist splint. The splint immobilizes the wrist in a neutral position to decrease bending and compression of the nerve. Persistent symptoms or hand weakness may be an indication for surgery to relieve the pressure on the median nerve.

## Peripheral Neuropathy

Some patients with Sjogren's syndrome develop a peripheral neuropathy. The process is characterized by an injury to one or more of the peripheral nerves in the legs and arms, and may target either sensory or motor nerve fibers, or both. The damage occurs either from a direct assault on the nerve tissue by the immune system or from vasculitis (vessel inflammation) causing interruption of the nerve's blood supply.

A sensory peripheral neuropathy, the most common type in Sjogren's syndrome, is usually symmetrical (involves limbs on both sides of the body) and mild. It causes numbness, tingling, burning, and, less commonly, difficulties with balance and manual dexterity. A physical examination will generally reveal an area of abnormal sensation in the legs and arms with a "stocking and glove" distribution.

A motor peripheral neuropathy results in muscle weakness and impairs the body's movements. The examination may show absent reflexes or a wrist or foot drop. The loss of muscle strength due to neuropathy is a serious but rare complication of Sjogren's syndrome. The information from a medical history and a physical examination may be adequate for the diagnosis of neurological problems. However, laboratory and special studies may be necessary to corroborate the physician's initial impressions. For example, in cases of suspected peripheral neuropathy, electromyography and nerve conduction velocity tests are often obtained to determine the precise extent and severity of peripheral nerve damage.

The goal in treating a sensory peripheral neuropathy is to reduce the symptoms of intense pain and burning. Significant or progressive weakness due to a motor neuropathy may be an indication for treatment with steroids or other potent medications that suppress the immune system.

### Cranial Neuropathy

The cranial nerves may also be affected in Sjogren's syndrome. The best (and most common) example of such involvement is trigeminal neuropathy. The trigeminal nerve supplies sensation to the face and the surface of the eye (cornea), as well as nerve fibers to the organs of taste and smell. Damage to the trigeminal nerve can result in facial pain and diminished sensation, as well as loss of taste and smell.

### Central Nervous System Disorders

The central nervous system (CNS) is rarely involved in Sjogren's syndrome. A variety of signs and symptoms may occur, reflecting different areas of brain and spinal cord injury. In certain cases, the features of CNS disease in Sjogren's syndrome may resemble those seen in multiple sclerosis. Sophisticated testing and radiological procedures, including spinal fluid examination and brain magnetic resonance imaging scans, may be needed to evaluate the symptoms or signs of CNS problems.

# 13 Lymphoma in Sjogren's Syndrome

IN AUTOIMMUNE DISEASES such as Sjogren's syndrome, lymphocytes (white blood cells) attack and destroy organs and produce autoantibodies (antibodies to these organs). While these attacks are certainly destructive, misguided, and without reason, the lymphocytes responsible are benign and lack any features of the lymphoid malignancy called lymphoma. In other Sjogren's syndrome patients, however, this is not the case.

Approximately 5 percent of Sjogren's syndrome patients develop enlarged lymph nodes (usually in the neck, groin, or armpit) or other symptoms suggesting a possible lymphoma. Biopsy of the lymph nodes is performed and may show only benign reactive lymphocytes, as expected in patients with autoimmune diseases. Sometimes it is difficult to tell whether the cells are benign, malignant, or something in between, a condition called pseudolymphoma. The term pseudolymphoma is used when the tissue lesions show tumor-like aggregates of lymphoid cells but fail to meet the histologic criteria for malignancy. A consultation with experienced lymph node pathologists may be invaluable in such cases. Molecular, biological, and immunological techniques can determine at the DNA or protein level whether the lymphocytes in question contain a single molecular population (i.e., are monoclonal, representing a single, dominant clone of cells) or a varied population (oligo or polyclonal). This can be helpful because a single clone favors a diagnosis of lymphoma. The true lymphomas are often classified as non-Hodgkin's lymphomas. Others are associated with monoclonal immunoglobulin M and resemble Waldenstrom's macroglobulinemia.

Even if a single clone is found, it may never evolve to a rapidly expanding and therefore more dangerous population of lymphocytes. Thus, some patients with Sjogren's syndrome may not need immediate treatment but can be followed closely (what doctors call watchful waiting) to determine whether the lymphoma remains localized or becomes more extensive. Because decisions about treatment are sometimes difficult and complex, the opinion of a cancer specialist, or oncologist, can be invaluable. Since lymphoma in Sjogren's syndrome is relatively rare, no single physician has had a great deal of experience with this problem; therefore, a team approach is best.

In pseudolymphoma, the site of lymphoproliferation determines the clinical appearance. Striking regional lymphadenopathy (enlargement of the lymph nodes) may be the predominant clinical feature. On the other hand, lymphoid infiltration may be excessive in only one organ far from the salivary or lacrimal glands, such as the kidney or lung. These organs may become functionally impaired, resulting in renal abnormalities or pulmonary insufficiency.

Features that should alert the clinician to the possibility of extra-glandular lymphoproliferation (increase in lymphoid tissue) in a patient with Sjogren's syndrome are regional or generalized node swelling, enlarged liver or spleen, lung infiltrates, kidney abnormalities, skin lesions, low white blood cell count, and elevated gamma globulins. Vasculitis (vessel inflammation) may be present, but arthritis (joint inflammation) is rare in such patients. Pseudolymphoma cannot be clearly defined, but it occupies the middle portion of a spectrum (Table 8) that includes benign disease, on the one hand, and frankly malignant disease, on the other.

Lymphocytes are divided into two major classes, called T cells and B cells. The T cells mediate delayed hypersensitive and cellular immunity (e.g., the skin test for tuberculosis). The B cells make gamma globulins (called immunoglobulin), antibodies (specific immunoglobulins), and abnormal antibodies (called antoantibodies, such as Ro/SS-A and La/SS-B). (The lymphocytes in lymphoma are almost invariably B cells.) This suggests that the same process and factors that lead to autoimmune disease may also be involved in malignancy. Perhaps the lymphoma is an

---

**TABLE 8   THE SPECTRUM OF SJOGREN'S SYNDROME**

| Benign Autoimmune Exocrinopathy | Pseudolymphoma | Malignant Lymphoma |
|---|---|---|
| *Clinical* | | |
| Xerostomia* | Lymphadenopathy | Massive lymphadenopathy |
| Xerophthalmia[†] | Splenomegaly[§] | Massive salivary gland enlargement |
| Rheumatoid arthritis (or another systemic rheumatic disease) | Purpura[‖] Pulmonary infiltrates Renal infiltrates | Wasting |
| *Pathology* | | |
| Benign lymphoid infiltrates confined to glandular tissue | Atypical extraglandular lymphoid infiltrates | B-cell lymphoma |
| **Serology** | | |
| Hypergammaglobulinemia[‡] Anti-Ro and -La (+) | Hypergammaglobulinemia Anti-Ro and -La (+) Monoclonal spike | Hypogammaglobulinemia** Loss of autoantibodies |

\* Dry mouth.
[†] Dry eyes.
[‡] Increased level of immunoglobulins in the blood.
[§] Enlarged spleen.
[‖] Hemorrhage into the skin.
\*\* Decreased level of immunoglobulins in the blood.

ultimate step in the chain of immunopathological events starting with autoimmunity.

Cancer researchers now recognize that a failure of apoptosis (programmed cell death) is a major contributing factor in malignancy. Many anticancer drugs work by overcoming this defect in apoptosis. There is now evidence of defective lymphocyte apoptosis in Sjogren's syndrome as well, as discussed in Chapter 1. Thus, an abnormality of apoptosis seems to be an important unifying feature of both autoimmune and lymphoid malignant disease in Sjogren's syndrome.

**Thomas T. Provost, MD**

# 14 The Skin and Sjogren's Syndrome

SJOGREN'S SYNDROME IS a systemic disease, and one of the organs commonly involved is the skin. The most common skin manifestation of Sjogren's syndrome is dryness. There is evidence, although incomplete, that the glands in the skin responsible for producing moisture (sweat and sebaceous glands) are affected. Generalized dryness of the skin occurs in as many as 50 percent of Sjogren's syndrome patients. The skin, instead of being soft and smooth, is rough. If the dryness is severe, cracking and fissuring of the skin can occur. These fissures easily become secondarily infected, producing red, itchy areas.

At times, the only manifestation of dryness is itchy skin. Scratching of the skin, if vigorous, can produce excoriations that can become secondarily infected. Many times, however, repeated scratching causes the pigment cells in the outer layer of the skin to become very active, resulting in darkening at the site of scratching. This increased pigmentation can occur at sites of previous low-grade infections (i.e., previous fissures or excoriations). It is transient and will end following the disappearance of the low-grade infection and scratching of the skin.

Skin dryness is worse during the wintertime in the northern latitudes. With the onset of winter, humidity decreases with temperature. This added burden of low humidity aggravates the already dry skin of a Sjogren's syndrome patient. Itching, cracking and fissuring, excoriations, low-grade infections, and increased pigmentation at sites of trauma are generally more prominent in the wintertime.

In marked contrast, the summer months are associated with increased humidity, and the skin dryness associated with Sjogren's syndrome is generally less prominent. Sjogren's syndrome patients living year round in dry areas such as the mountain states and the Southwest may experience continued skin problems. By contrast, patients living in warm, moist areas such as South Florida and the Gulf states generally have far less trouble with their skin.

Treatment of severe dryness of the skin (xerosis) involves occluding (covering) the skin to trap normal sweat and sebaceous gland secretions on the skin before they evaporate. This involves the application of creams and ointments (heavier than creams) to the affected areas frequently (three or four times a day). The creams and ointments occlude the skin and promote hydration. Lotions are much lighter than creams and ointments. They evaporate quickly and aggravate skin dryness; therefore, they should not be used to treat dryness in patients with Sjogren's syndrome.

According to my patients, an effective form of therapy is to shower for no longer than 5 minutes, pat the skin dry (leaving a small residue of moisture), and then apply an occlusive ointment such as Eucerin or Aquaphor, especially to areas of previous itching.

In addition to the frequent use of creams and ointments, as well as the bathing regimen, patients should be cautioned to avoid frequent bathing because normal body oils are depleted by bathing and soaps. Soaps with a high content of emollients (e.g., Dove, Camay) are highly recommended. Cetaphil, a soap substitute, and Basis soap are also of value.

For patients living in the northern climates, the humidity of the home can be increased to comfort the itchy skin of Sjogren's syndrome patients. A humidifier attached to the furnace or placed in the bedroom is very effective in providing increased humidity (the bedroom is the room in which an individual spends the most time each day, hence the desirability of having a humidifier there). In addition, large, leafy plants that must be frequently watered create a greenhouse effect, increasing the humidity.

These measures have proven very successful in the treatment of patients with itchy, dry skin. At times, topical steroid creams and ointments, but not lotions, are also effective. Topical steroids have an anti-itch effect.

## Raynaud's Phenomenon

About 20 percent of patients with Sjogren's syndrome have a classic triphasic color response to exposure to cold. There is an initial sharply demarcated blanching (whitening) of the fingers or toes upon cold exposure. Then, with rewarming, there is an initial bluish coloration followed by generalized redness. Pain is commonly present, especially during the rewarming phase (see Chapter 9).

## Other Skin Lesions Associated with Sjogren's Syndrome

In recent years, Sjogren's syndrome patients with anti-Ro(SS-A) antibodies (approximately 30 percent of a lip biopsy-positive outpatient Sjogren's syndrome population seen by internists, allergists, gynecologists, and dermatologists) have been shown to develop, on occasion, a photosensitive (light-sensitive) cutaneous (skin) disease. These patients develop either annular (ring-like) red lesions generally involving the arms, trunk, and back, with little involvement of the face, or red, scaly lesions resembling psoriasis with the same distribution. These skin lesions are identical to those seen in patients who have subacute cutaneous lupus erythematosus, a rather benign form of cutaneous lupus.

Anti-Ro(SS-A) antibody-positive Sjogren's syndrome patients who develop the lesions of subacute cutaneous lupus erythematosus are generally very sensitive to the sun. Many of these patients burn from sunlight passing through the windshield of a car or through window glass. This means that relatively low-energy ultraviolet light, which at most will produce only darkening of the skin over a prolonged period of time in normal individuals, will produce acute, red, sometimes painful lesions in these patients.

It is recommended that anti-Ro(SS-A) antibody-positive Sjogren's syndrome patients avoid excessive sun exposure and judiciously apply sunscreens [with sun protective factor (SPF) 15] half an hour before going outdoors. Some anti-Ro(SS-A) antibody-positive Sjogren's syndrome patients may develop a photosensitive dermatitis after having had only Sjogren's syndrome for many years.

The dermatitis of subacute cutaneous lupus erythematosus generally responds to hydroxychloroquine, topical steroids, or diaminodiphenylsulfone.

Japanese investigators have recently reported the development of a raised, erythematous, plaque-like lesion with central clearing in some of their anti-Ro(SS-A) antibody-positive Sjogren's syndrome patients. This donut-like lesion appears to be uniquely associated with Japanese patients. Similar lesions have not been detected in American patients with Sjogren's syndrome, regardless of race.

In addition to the lesions of subacute cutaneous lupus erythematosus, Sjogren's syndrome patients, especially those possessing anti-Ro(SS-A) antibodies, are at risk to develop lesions of cutaneous vasculitis. Two forms of cutaneous vasculitis occur. The most common are erythematous palpable and non-palpable lesions on the lower extremities. Necrosis and small ulcerations may occur.

The second type of vasculitic lesion resembles urticaria (hives). Unlike common hives, which come and go over a 6-hour period, these urticaria-like lesions persist for days. Small hemorrhage dots may appear in the lesion (petechiae) indicative of damage to blood vessels in the lesion. A peculiar burning sensation, especially with the application of light pressure to the lesion, is common.

The presence of these vasculitic lesions may indicate the presence of systemic vasculitis, which the physician must evaluate.

Treatment of the vasculitis is variable. If no systemic features are detected, no therapy may be an option or the patient may be treated with hydroxychloroquine or diaminodiphenylsulfone.

If systemic features of vasculitis are detected or if necrosis and ulcerations are extensive, corticosteroids and/or immunosuppressive agents (Azathioprine, Cytoxan) may be indicated.

### Hair

Some Sjogren's syndrome patients describe having lusterless, dull hair. This problem has not been studied, but full-body shampoos (e.g., Johnson and Johnson's Baby Shampoo) and/or conditioners that replace hair oils may prove beneficial.

At times following a severe illness, Sjogren's syndrome patients may experience transient hair loss (alopecia). Normally growing hairs, termed anagen, pass into a resting phase, termed telogen, when illness occurs. This process, occurring over a 3-month period, results in loss of the original hair, which is replaced by new hair. At times, with a chronic illness and/or the use of immunosuppressive drugs, this transient hair loss may become dramatic. However, in general with the restoration of health, the alopecia subsides and normal hair growth resumes.

## General Principles of Skin Care

Sjogren's syndrome patients in general have a tendency toward dryness. This is exacerbated during the wintertime or in dry climates. Unscented moisturizers applied to the skin should be liberally used. Scented moisturizers contain alcohols and aldehydes as perfumes, which tend to dry the skin. Lotions are to be avoided, as are such cosmetic preparations as Retin-A cream and facial astringents (because of their drying effect).

Itching is a prominent complaint in Sjogren's syndrome patients, especially those with very dry skin. Potent topical steroids should be used with caution. Overusage of these drugs for their anti-itch effect can produce thinning of the skin. Increased hydration of the skin alone, using moisturizers, may produce the same beneficial effect. Where possible, antihistamines, because of their drying effect on mucous membranes, should be avoided in treating the itchy skin of Sjogren's syndrome patients.

Finally, warm, moist home conditions produced by the use of humidifiers and large, leafy plants are of great benefit. Extremes of cold and dryness are to be avoided because they reduce hydration of the skin and trigger Raynaud's phenomenon.

# 15 Allergy and Sjogren's Syndrome

THE PATIENT WHO is eventually diagnosed as having Sjogren's syndrome often appears first in an allergist's office. This is not surprising since many of the symptoms of Sjogren's syndrome initially resemble those of allergic reactions. Red, irritated eyes, a dry mouth, sore throat, and stuffy ears and nose, all unexplained by infection, may make a patient suspect allergies. Moreover, during the winter months, the symptoms get worse with exposure to the drying effect of central heating.

Since as many as 10 percent of the general population have allergies, a patient can have both Sjogren's syndrome and allergies. When performing a medical workup on a patient who is eventually diagnosed with Sjogren's syndrome, the allergist will find no association between the symptoms and possible exposure to or ingestion of an allergenic substance. Sjogren's syndrome patients usually do not complain of sneezing or of itchy eyes and nose. Because of their drying side effects, antihistamines may well have made the symptoms of these patients worse.

Skin tests for allergies to foods or inhalants will be negative in the patient with Sjogren's syndrome. A blood test for the presence of immunoglobin E (IgE), a blood protein that is usually elevated in allergic persons, will be within normal limits. Even if allergies are found, an antinuclear antibody (ANA) test should be ordered for any patient who has symptoms of Sjogren's syndrome.

When allergies coexist with Sjogren's syndrome, treatment is fraught with difficulty. The best medication for one disorder may be contraindicated in the other. Close interaction between the various treating physicians is mandatory.

## What Causes Allergies?

Allergic persons are normal except for the over-production of IgE. This can be measured by a sensitive blood test. An elevated measurement indicates an increased susceptibility to allergic disease.

The symptoms of allergy result from the release of certain chemicals, such as histamine, within the body. These chemicals are stored in cells, called basophils and mast cells, which are found even in those who are not allergic. In allergic individuals, proteins in foods or the environment, called allergens, cause allergic reactions.

## Allergic Reactions

An allergic reaction occurs when all three components—mast cells, IgE, and an allergen—are present at the same time. Allergic reactions may manifest as skin rashes; chest wheezing; itchy, stuffy nose and ears; post-nasal drip; or itching, irritated eyes. This can be a seasonal problem if an individual is allergic to environmental allergens, such as trees, grass, molds, or weeds, or a perennial problem if the allergen is dust, animals, or foods.

## Testing for Allergies

Testing for allergies is done in two ways. The more sensitive method is to place a small quantity of the suspected allergen just under the skin with a syringe. If the individual is allergic to the material, a local reaction of redness, itching, and a small swelling will occur within 15 minutes.

A second way of testing for specific allergies is to test the patient's blood with RAST tests. The RAST test measures the quantity of IgE in the blood that is specific for a particular allergen. These tests are not as sensitive as skin tests and may be more costly but may be especially useful for young patients (under 4 years of age), who often cannot sit still for skin testing, or for patients who cannot be taken off antihistamines.

## Avoiding Exposure to Allergens

The mainstay of allergic treatment is avoiding exposure to known allergens. A person who is allergic to animals, for example, should avoid them as much as possible. Very often, just removing the animal from the bedroom will lessen the symptoms.

It is possible to be allergic to one breed of animal and not another. For instance, an allergic reaction to a German shepherd in one person's house may not happen in another house with a Doberman pinscher. One could be allergic to a horse and not other animals. Because dog allergens are found in dander, urine, and saliva, all dogs can produce allergies in susceptible persons. There is no such thing as a nonallergenic dog. The same holds true for cats.

To avoid exposure to animal allergens, one must avoid objects consisting of animal substances, such as mattresses made of hog or horse hair; pillows, comforters, and furniture containing feathers; and carpet linings consisting of cow's hair.

To reduce house dust, a major allergen, the most important room to keep clean is the bedroom, where one ordinarily spends a good deal of time. To facilitate cleaning, the bedroom should be kept as simple as possible, with wood floors, no curtains, little stuffed furniture, and few books and toys. Cleaning daily with a vacuum cleaner, which will remove the dust, is better than shuffling the dust around the room with a cloth.

House mites, microscopic bugs that are a major component of dust, live off human skin. This unique diet means that they are often found in bedding areas, since this is where most people spend a great deal of time. Special mattress and pillow covers that prevent mites from accumulating in bedding are available.

Molds, consisting of microscopic organisms that tend to grow in damp and poorly lit areas, are another source of allergic exposure. Easily identified, the blackish-greenish material is often found on shower curtains or in damp basements. Individuals whose allergies are exacerbated on damp days are often allergic to molds. Once present, molds are hard to eradicate. Cleaning with antifungal agents, bleach, or ammonia helps to destroy them. To remove mold, change the environment—increase aeration of the area, open windows or doors, or remove the dampness with a dehumidifier or by sealing leaks. Chemicals are often added to wallpaper paste to prevent mold buildup behind wallpaper.

Perfume, smoke, chemicals, dry air, and other environmental irritants that exacerbate allergic symptoms should be avoided by patients with either Sjogren's syndrome or allergic disease. In some individuals, symptoms worsen with acute changes in barometric pressure or temperature. Knowing that these physical factors can make things worse helps allergic individuals to reduce their symptoms by avoiding exposure.

Wide-lens, wraparound goggles offer practical protection from allergens such as pollen, mold, dander, and dust. These goggles can be obtained as sun goggles or as clear goggles that can be worn indoors. A mask may also be worn on bad allergy days to reduce exposure to allergens.

## Allergy Treatments

The best treatment is to avoid the suspected allergen. Because allergens such as grass, weeds, and house dust cannot be completely avoided, treatment with medications may be necessary. These medications include decongestants, antihistamines, and corticosteroids. Only the antihistamines are contraindicated in a person with Sjogren's syndrome because they tend to cause dryness—the last thing a Sjogren's syndrome patient wants. However, some of the newer antihistamines may be used if necessary and if given in a sufficiently low dosage.

Patients may obtain symptomatic relief from allergic eye symptoms with the use of eye drops, which are available by prescription from an ophthalmologist or optometrist. Some drops may be used continuously, when necessary to prevent eye allergies and will not dry out the eyes. Patients should work closely with their healthcare specialist to find an eye preparation to treat both allergic symptoms and Sjogren's syndrome.

For the patient with allergies affecting the nose and sinuses, there are many medications that will relieve symptoms. These consist of oral decongestants and nasal sprays that contain either corticosteroids or other anti-inflammatories (e.g., sodium cromolyn). Neither of these types of nasal sprays is absorbed by the body.

Since the asthmatic patient should not be dried out, most medications used to treat asthma are well tolerated by the patient with Sjogren's syndrome.

Allergic skin rashes can be treated with topical or oral corticosteroids. Newer topical antihistamines avoid the problem of making a patient allergic as a result of applying the antihistamine to the skin.

Allergy shots also help sufferers. Improvement occurs over several years as the dosage of the shots is increased. This form of therapy should be reserved for patients whose allergic symptoms are not helped by medications or whose symptoms exist for a prolonged period of time, such as more than 3 weeks a year.

# 16 Fibromyalgia Complicating Sjogren's Syndrome

OVER THE LAST FEW YEARS, there has been an increasing realization that many patients with Sjogren's syndrome have an additional problem: fibromyalgia. It is important for patients and their doctors to differentiate between symptoms due to Sjogren's syndrome itself and those due to fibromyalgia, as the treatments are often quite different. Furthermore, the treatment of some features of fibromyalgia may make the symptoms of Sjogren's syndrome worse and vice versa.

## What Is Fibromyalgia?

Fibromyalgia is not a new disease. It was once called fibrositis, a term first used by Sir William Gowers, an English physician, when giving a lecture on lumbago in 1904. At that time, it was thought that fibrositis was due to inflammation of fibrous tissue between muscle bundles. This is now known to be incorrect. For this reason, the term fibrositis was abandoned and the name fibromyalgia officially adopted by the American College of Rheumatology in 1990.

The basic symptom of fibromyalgia is chronic, widespread pain. Many patients also have tender skin. Most patients believe that their pain arises from muscle, but many also have a feeling of swelling in their soft tissues close to joints. This may lead to an incorrect diagnosis of arthritis. A flare of fibromyalgia in a patient with Sjogren's syndrome may be mistaken for increased activity of Sjogren's syndrome itself. The pain of fibromyalgia typically waxes and wanes in intensity. Flares are often associated with unaccustomed exertion, lack of sleep, cold exposure, soft tissue injuries, and psychological stress. Although most fibromyalgia patients have widespread body pain, there are often a few locations that are the major foci of pain. These pain centers characteristically shift to other locations, often in response to injuries or biomechanical stresses.

Most patients with widespread pain fitting this description have multiple tender areas in their muscles. A tender area (or tender point, as it is usually called) is the core physical finding of the fibromyalgia syndrome. Although there are multiple tender point areas, physicians palpate 9 paired tender points (i.e., 18 in total). A diagnosis of fibromyalgia can be confidently made if the patient has 11 or more tender areas in association with a history of widespread pain.

For most patients, fibromyalgia is more than a muscle pain problem; they typically have an array of other symptoms. For instance, nearly all fibromyalgia patients have severe fatigue, poor sleep, and postexertional pain. Other common symptoms include tension headaches, cold intolerance, fluid retention, jaw pain, dizziness, low-grade depression, and numbness and tingling in the extremities. Many fibromyalgia patients, with or without associated Sjogren's syndrome, also complain of dry mouth and dry eyes. Furthermore, patients with fibromyalgia have an increased prevalence of other readily recognized syndromes, such as irritable bowel (spastic colon), irritable bladder, migraine headaches, premenstrual syndrome, Raynaud's phenomenon, and restless leg syndrome. Many patients with fibromyalgia also have symptoms of Sjogren's syndrome. This overlap in the symptoms between the two syndromes often confuses both patients and doctors.

## How Is Fibromyalgia Related to Sjogren's Syndrome?

One report in the literature states that 50 percent of Scandinavian patients with Sjogren's syndrome also have fibromyalgia. No comparable studies have been done on North American patients. Although most patients with Sjogren's syndrome have a well-established diagnosis, there may be some patients with a diagnosis of fibromyalgia in whom the Sjogren's syndrome has gone unrecognized. One recent study found several new cases of Sjogren's syndrome in a group of 72 fibromyalgia patients who were screened with Schirmer's test and minor salivary gland lip biopsies. The association of fibromyalgia with Sjogren's syndrome is not unique. About 40 percent of patients with systemic lupus erythematosus also develop fibromyalgia, as do 25 percent of patients with rheumatoid arthritis. It is now apparent that fibromyalgia may be the end result of many chronic pain states and other chronic illnesses. Some patients with chronic infectious diseases, such as Lyme disease and human immunodeficiency virus infection, also show an increased tendency to develop fibromyalgia. Recently, an association between hepatitis C infection and fibromyalgia has been described. Interestingly, hepatitis C has also been linked to Sjogren's syndrome in some patients. The association of fibromyalgia with Sjogren's syndrome is thus part of a spectrum of overlap that is increasingly being recognized in patients with other rheumatic disorders.

The prevalence of fibromyalgia in the U.S. population has recently been estimated from an epidemiological study in Wichita. The overall prevalence is estimated to be 2 percent. Fibromyalgia occurs more commonly in women, in whom the prevalence is 3.4 percent compared to 0.5 percent in men. There is a linear increase in fibromyalgia symptoms in the general population from the late teens up to the seventh decade. Approximately 7.5 percent of women can be expected to have fibromyalgia symptoms by the time they reach the age of 80. The proportion of these patients who also have Sjogren's syndrome is not currently known.

## The Consequences of Fibromyalgia

Chronic musculoskeletal pain, whether it arises from arthritis or from muscle in fibromyalgia or the joints in Sjogren's syndrome, often impairs the patient's quality of life. Fibromyalgia patients also have a sleep disorder characterized by frequent awakenings and fragmented sleep. This leads to fatigue. The combination of chronic muscular pain and fatigue means that most Sjogren's/fibromyalgia patients need more time to get started in the morning and often require extra rest periods during the day. They have difficulty with tasks that demand repetitive or sustained muscle action and often need frequent time-outs to complete even menial tasks. Activities that may be well tolerated for short periods of time become aggravating when carried out for long periods. Prolonged muscular activity, especially under stress or in uncomfortable climatic conditions, seems to aggravate the muscle pain of fibromyalgia. In general, most patients with fibromyalgia have to make lifestyle adaptations to minimize their discomfort. This often has a negative impact on vocational and avocational activities as well as on marriage and other relationships. Currently, there is no cure for fibromyalgia, and long-term follow-up studies show that the symptoms persist for many years.

## Treatment of Fibromyalgia Symptoms

In general, medications are not helpful in controlling the muscle pain experienced by fibromyalgia patients. For instance, nonsteroidal medications such as Ibuprofen may take the edge off the pain but are seldom more than 20 percent effective. Corticosteroids, such as prednisone, are not helpful. This is an important distinction, as some patients with Sjogren's syndrome develop muscle inflammation (myositis), which is helped by treatment with corticosteroids. However, corticosteroids may aggravate fibromyalgia symptoms. For instance, long-term corticosteroid use may cause muscle weakness and exacerbate fibromyalgia. High-dose corticosteroids commonly cause a sleep disturbance; this aggravates the already fragmented sleep of the fibromyalgia patient. Narcotic analgesics may provide pain relief but should be used sparingly and only for short periods of time; they will often aggravate dryness of the eyes and mouth, as well as causing constipation.

The accumulating experience of treating patients with fibromyalgia indicates that there are three essential components that need to be addressed.

### Sleep

If the fragmented sleep of fibromyalgia is improved, there seems to be a worthwhile improvement in muscle pain. It is important for physicians to analyze the sleep disturbance to rule out potentially treatable conditions such as sleep apnea, tooth grinding, and restless leg syndrome. Most fibromyalgia patients are helped by low dosages of drugs that are usually used to treat depression, the so-called tricyclic antidepressants; common examples include amitriptyline, doxepin, trazedone, and nortriptyline. It should be stressed that the dosages needed to treat sleep are much less than those used to treat depression. However, there is a potential problem in patients with Sjogren's syndrome, as many of these drugs tend to cause dry mouth. Hence, the tricyclic medications are often unacceptable to patients with Sjogren's syndrome. It is often necessary to use more conventional tranquilizers and sleeping medications such as alprazolam and zolpidem or over-the-counter sleep aids such as diphenhydramine.

### Exercise

The second major component in treating fibromyalgia is exercise. Indeed, there is a strong consensus that *patients with fibromyalgia cannot afford not to exercise*. However, muscle pain and severe fatigue are powerful excuses for not exercising. All Sjogren's syndrome patients with symptoms of fibromyalgia need to develop a home program of muscle stretching, gentle strengthening, and aerobic conditioning. There are several points that should be stressed about exercise in Sjogren's syndrome patients with associated fibromyalgia:

1   Exercise means health training, not sports training. It should not be competitive or directed toward a single point in time, rather it must be lifelong.

2   Exercise should be nonimpact loading (e.g. walking rather than running).

3   Anaerobic exercise should be done three or four times a week at about 70 percent of the maximum pulse rate for 20–30 minutes. You can calculate your theoretical maximum pulse rate by subtracting your age from 220. Thus, if you are 50, your maximum pulse rate is 170, and you should aim to raise it to 119 beats per minute (i.e., 70 percent of 170) with exercise. Exercises that are suitable for raising the pulse rate include fast walking and the use of a stationary exercycle or NordicTrak.

4   Regular exercise needs to become part of the patient's lifestyle, not something that is indulged in for 3–6 months.

Stretching exercises are best taught by a physical therapist or exercise physiologist. Patients who are very deconditioned or incapacitated are often helped by starting out with water therapy using a buoyancy belt (Aqua-Jogger). Those patients who adopt a regular exercise program soon appreciate its benefits and make it a lifestyle priority, not an afterthought.

## Myofascial Therapy

The third component of treating muscle pain in fibromyalgia is specific muscle therapy (myofascial therapy). Many patients get short-term relief from physical modalities such as passive stretching, massage, heat treatment, and acupuncture. Doctors specializing in rehabilitation medicine and rheumatology often inject tender point areas with a local anesthetic such as Procaine or Lidocaine. It should be noted that these are not cortisone injections. In my experience, about 80 percent of fibromyalgia patients benefit from such injections, which may make their exercise routine more effective. Trigger point therapy should be tried when there is a major focus of pain in just one or two areas. It is evident that total body injections cannot be given. Procaine in a total volume of 10 cc or more often makes patients feel dizzy; this is the main reason for restricting it to major pain foci. Some patients are allergic to local anesthetics, and the use of such injections could cause life-threatening reactions. Always tell your doctor if you have such allergies. The relief of pain experienced from expertly performed trigger point injections often lasts for 2 to 6 months. This period should be used as an opportunity to promote the exercise program.

## Conclusion

Fibromyalgia and Sjogren's syndrome are chronic problems for which there are currently no cures. These conditions often severely affect the patient's quality of life. There is considerable overlap in the symptoms of the two conditions. However, Sjogren's syndrome is an autoimmune disease, whereas fibromyalgia is not. This distinctive difference in the underlying disease mechanisms means that the treatment options are also different. One of the most important steps that patients with Sjogren's syndrome can take, whether or not they have fibromyalgia, is to become more medically educated and aware of the treatment options and their potential complications. In reading this book, you are taking a major step down that educational highway.

# Gynecology
## and Pregnancy

John J. Willems, MD,

Lila Nachtigall, MD

# 17 Gynecological Issues in Women with Sjogren's Syndrome

WHEN A RHEUMATOLOGIST or primary healthcare provider refers a woman with Sjogren's syndrome to a gynecologist for evaluation, her problem is usually vaginal dryness and dyspareunia (painful intercourse), caused by lack of natural lubrication. Other common causes for gynecological referral in women with Sjogren's syndrome are yeast infections and vulvar (external) discomfort.

Many women with Sjogren's syndrome do have adequate vaginal lubrication. On the other hand, vaginal dryness, vulvar discomfort, and yeast infections are common problems in women who do not have Sjogren's syndrome. Thus, these conditions are not always related to dry eyes and dry mouth. The first step in the gynecological examination is to rule out other causes of these symptoms.

Although many women with Sjogren's syndrome are no longer interested in bearing children, questions do arise concerning Sjogren's syndrome and obstetrical risks. These will be considered separately in Chapters 18 and 19.

Women at the other end of the reproductive age range have a great interest in and concern about estrogen replacement therapy. This concern is not only about estrogen in general but also about the effect of estrogen on Sjogren's syndrome in particular. In this chapter, estrogen replacement therapy will be reviewed, along with nonhormonal lubricants, management of yeast infections, and new directions in gynecological research for women with Sjogren's syndrome.

## Special Problems in Women with Sjogren's Syndrome

Sjogren's syndrome is not the uncommon problem that many have been taught to believe. This disorder, including primary Sjogren's syndrome and Sjogren's syndrome in association with other autoimmune diseases, may be the second most common rheumatological disease in the United States. Up to 30 percent of patients with rheumatoid arthritis, 10 percent of those with systemic lupus erythematosus, and 1 percent of those with scleroderma have secondary Sjogren's syndrome. No one understands why Sjogren's syndrome affects predominantly women or why it tends to occur in the fourth decade of life or later. Also, the incidence of gynecological problems in women with Sjogren's syndrome is not known with certainty, although, as noted above, some degree of vaginal dryness, vulvar discomfort, or vaginal yeast infection is common.

Strictly speaking, natural vaginal lubrication primarily involves a fluid derived from the bloodstream across the vaginal walls and is unrelated to the moisture-producing function of the exocrine glands like the salivary or lacrimal (tear) glands that are so prominently affected by Sjogren's syndrome. Therefore, any increase in vaginal dryness in women with Sjogren's syndrome beyond that associated with estrogen deficiency or vaginal infection may be related to an underlying autoimmune effect of Sjogren's syndrome on the vascular supply to the vagina. Alternatively, the stress of chronic illness tends to reduce vaginal moisture, and this effect may be the operant cause.

In addition to the fact that women with Sjogren's syndrome can have special obstetrical and gynecological problems, very little has been written about those problems. In a recent computer search of the medical literature over the last 5 years, no articles were found on the treatment of dyspareunia (painful sexual relations) and Sjogren's syndrome.

### Ruling Out Other Causes

Before the gynecologist can attribute vaginal dryness to Sjogren's syndrome, other causes must be ruled out. At menopause, for example, decreased estrogen levels may lead to vaginal symptoms such as dryness and pain with intercourse, which can also happen when a woman has her ovaries (the predominant source of estrogen) surgically removed.

Vaginal infections can cause discomfort during or after intercourse. Chronic illnesses such as diabetes or lupus may cause loss of lubrication due to the debilitating nature of the disease, loss of sexual interest, or both.

Medications such as antidepressants, antihistamines, and cardiac and blood pressure medications can affect both sexual response and vaginal lubrication.

Normal aging affects the rapidity of production and the quantity of vaginal lubrication.

Prior painful intercourse can inhibit lubrication when the woman anticipates another painful experience. Lack of adequate sexual stimulation, for whatever reason, can be related to limited lubrication. Lastly, pelvic pathology (i.e., ovarian tumors, uterine fibroids) can cause painful intercourse and vaginal dryness secondarily.

## Treatment of Gynecological Problems in Sjogren's Syndrome Patients

Once other causes of vaginal dryness and painful coitus have been investigated and ruled out, a true relationship to Sjogren's syndrome may be inferred. The patient and her partner need to be reassured that this is a physiological problem and is not related to a failure of sexual arousal.

To replace or supplement natural vaginal lubrication, sterile, greaseless lubricants are helpful. One must be careful when it comes to advertising and vaginal preparations. Madison Avenue has a tendency to tout certain products as "personal lubricants" with overtones of enhanced sexual fulfillment. However, any lubricant with a color, taste, or any other additive is not the right one for most women and is definitely not appropriate for vaginal dryness related to Sjogren's syndrome.

The ideal lubricant is colorless, odorless, tasteless, water-soluble, and of a consistency that allows it to remain in the vagina. If too much lubricant is used, the result is frictionless and rather messy coitus. If this is a persistent problem, a woman might consider using a small amount of vaginal gel or cream and then adding a thin layer directly to her partner's penis.

It is important to note the difference between a vaginal lubricant and a vaginal moisturizer. A lubricant should be used only for intercourse or other vaginal sexual activity. Currently, there are a large number of acceptable lubricants from which to choose. Moisturizers, available over the counter, are for regular use to attract liquid to the dry vaginal area. Both lubricants and moisturizers have a very acidic pH that helps fight vaginal infections, but therefore might be irritating to the partner. Patients using some moisturizers should be aware that they can leave a white residue that can be confused with a yeast infection.

Only water-soluble lubricants should be used in the vagina; oil-based lubricants foil the vagina's natural self-cleansing mechanism. Oil-based lubricants are also fairly immune to douches. Moreover, they can trap natural moisture in the vagina and cause maceration of sensitive vaginal tissues. They have been implicated in some allergic problems. Because they impair sperm mobility, they are specifically contraindicated for the couple trying to conceive. Therefore, the internal use of preparations containing petrolatum or oils that seal in moisture, such as petroleum jelly or cocoa butter, is to be avoided.

Cortisone creams are not beneficial in this situation, and can further thin and sensitize tissues that are already very sensitive.

On the external vulvar surface, dryness may be treated with lubricating creams, as for other skin surfaces. Some women have reported that a light lubricating oil such as vitamin E oil is useful for vulvar skin.

When lack of lubrication is caused by decreased estrogen levels, whether due to natural or surgical menopause, correction is achieved with appropriate estrogen replacement.

Yeast infections are a common problem, particularly when a woman has a tendency toward diabetes, takes antibiotics, or has lost the protective effect of estrogen on the normal vaginal flora. They are also a problem in women with any immune system compromise, including those using steroid medications; this may cause the clinical perception that yeast infections are more common in Sjogren's syndrome. In addition, xerostomia (oral dryness) predisposes to oral yeast infection; increased vaginal dryness may have a similar effect.

Treatment of yeast infection first requires an accurate diagnosis. A telephone diagnosis is frequently inadequate. Treatment should be based on vaginal culture or microscopic analysis. Once the diagnosis is established, many curative treatments are available. Currently, over-the-counter products are very effective when used for the correctly diagnosed yeast infection. Prescription treatments include a one-dose vaginal treatment and fluconazole, a one-dose oral treatment. Other effective treatments include creams, topical gentian violet, and vaginal boric acid capsules. As a rule, vaginal creams are slightly more effective than vaginal suppositories because they provide more complete vaginal coverage.

When recurrent yeast infections are a problem, management of any underlying predisposition, such as control of blood sugar, is important. Ongoing recurrences may require a preventive program, such as one application of a vaginal treatment once a week or just before and after menses. This should be done only under a physician's direction and only after accurate diagnostic studies. Many women seen for chronic yeast infections and presumed failure of appropriate treatment are found no longer to have a yeast infection but rather persistent symptoms that feel like a yeast infection.

In summary, treatment of Sjogren's-related gynecological problems is symptomatic only. No cure has yet been found for the underlying disease. With personal testing and compassionate gynecological care, the Sjogren's syndrome patient can find what works best for her.

## Sjogren's Syndrome and Hormones

Women with Sjogren's syndrome often wonder if an autoimmune disease precludes the use of postmenopausal estrogen replacement therapy (ERT). As pointed out, estrogen taken orally or applied locally is very useful in combating postmenopausal vaginal dryness and painful intercourse. With regard to estrogen replacement in general, the clinical evidence is now fully convincing that blocking osteoporosis and reducing cardiovascular mortality while improving the quality of life by eliminating hot flashes and hormone-related vaginal dryness makes properly monitored ERT an overwhelmingly attractive management strategy. Recent findings have not only confirmed the markedly decreased risk of cardiovascular mortality but have also shown that the risk of Alzheimer's disease is lower among estrogen users compared to matched postmenopausal nonusers. If the woman has been taking estrogen for 7 or more years, the risk reduction is greater.

Earlier investigators were concerned that estrogen might have a negative influence on Sjogren's patients. It is still unknown why women are more prone to Sjogren's syndrome than men, but it is unlikely that the answer is estrogen alone. If estrogen were the culprit, Sjogren's flares might be seen during pregnancy, with its very high estrogen levels, and the incidence of the syndrome would not increase substantially just when a woman's estrogen production capacity is waning. The more plausible explanation is that a sex-linked immune dysfunction is responsible for the female preponderance. At Scripp's Clinic, we have not seen any increase in Sjogren's syndrome activity related to either ERT, oral contraceptive use, or pregnancy. In fact, overall data on connective tissue disorders suggest that a more likely time for a disease flare is just after delivery, when hormone levels are low. For this reason, we encourage adequate estrogen replacement for the properly screened postmenopausal Sjogren's syndrome patient.

For the most part, unless there is an underlying medical contraindication such as a personal history of breast cancer, active thrombophlebitis, or a history of thromboembolic disorders such as deep venous thrombosis or pulmonary embolus, estrogen/progestin replacement therapy is recommended for all postmenopausal patients.

For premenopausal Sjogren's syndrome patients, there are no specific contraindications to the use of low-dose oral contraceptives for birth control or menstrual cycle regulation aside from those that apply to all women, such as cigarette smoking and hypertension. Women who have the antiphospholipid antibody syndrome (see Chapter 19) must use extreme caution and consult their physician prior to using estrogen.

Although menopausal vaginal atrophy is worse in the Sjogren's syndrome patient, it still responds to local estrogen therapy, and only low doses are needed. A very simple way to note if the vagina needs estrogen is to test the pH (whether there is enough acidity) using pH paper, which can be purchased in the pharmacy. The goal is to have a reading of 5 or less. Even women taking oral or transdermal ERT may need to apply estrogen cream to the vagina once or twice a week. Within the next year, a slow-release estrogen ring should be available. This ring, placed in the vagina, releases a very tiny dose of estrogen to the vaginal tissues daily. It shows great promise as an excellent therapy for postmenopausal Sjogren's syndrome patients, whether or not they are taking ERT.

## New Directions for Gynecological Study in Sjogren's Syndrome

In the biomedical field, new questions are often raised faster than answers can be developed. Two new questions concerning Sjogren's syndrome patients are both in the area of hormone replacement.

Currently, there is great controversy in gynecology regarding the use of male hormones in addition to female hormones for the treatment of menopausal symptoms. Opinions range from sometimes to always to never. Potential benefits include an increase in energy, sense of well-being, libido, and sexual response. Potential complications include oily skin, acne, hair growth, water retention, and weight gain. This controversy affects Sjogren's syndrome patients because current research seems to indicate that added male hormone can increase tear production.

Also controversial is the possible superiority of one progestational agent over another. In general, if a woman has not had a hysterectomy, she is advised to replace both female hormones (estrogen and progesterone) at the time of menopause. This is done to protect the uterus from exposure to a continuous estrogen effect. Some investigators have suggested that natural oral micronized progesterone is superior to the commonly prescribed progesterone agent, especially for Sjogren's syndrome patients.

Both of these issues are unresolved and require further study. In probing further, we will be able to define more clearly the optimal hormone replacement program for the postmenopausal Sjogren's syndrome patient.

Jill P. Buyon, MD

# 18 Pregnancy in Women with Sjogren's Syndrome: Neonatal Problems

ANTIBODIES ARE AN essential part of the body's ability to protect itself against infection by foreign invaders such as bacteria and viruses. During the course of a healthy pregnancy, antibodies in the mother's circulation are transported across the placenta into the bloodstream of the developing fetus. The movement of maternal antibodies across the placenta begins at or around the end of the first trimester. The fetus is incapable of making antibodies on its own and is therefore completely dependent on maternal antibodies to fight infection. Unfortunately, the placenta cannot distinguish antibodies that are beneficial from those that might not be. Accordingly, for women with autoimmune diseases such as Sjogren's syndrome and systemic lupus erythematosus (SLE), abnormal antibodies directed against self molecules (autoantibodies, the hallmark of an autoimmune disease) can also cross the placenta and enter the fetal circulation.

The name given to fetal and neonatal illnesses caused by these antibodies is neonatal lupus. This term is extremely misleading. It originated because a skin rash initially seen in babies resembled that seen in adults with SLE. The first babies who were noted to have heart block were born to women who did have SLE. However, we now know that many mothers with affected children are themselves totally asymptomatic and only have the Sjogren's anti-SS-A/Ro and/or anti-SS-B/La antibodies in their blood (i.e., a mother who has anti-SS-A/Ro or SS-B/La antibodies and a child with neonatal lupus does not necessarily have Sjogren's syndrome or SLE). The child also does not have SLE but rather a disease acquired from the passage of maternal autoantibodies. Therefore, the name neonatal lupus is not accurate. Neonatal lupus is not a true systemic (multiple organ systems involved) disease.

### Fetal and Neonatal Problems

Autoantibodies vary widely, and specific autoantibodies, such as anti-SS-A/Ro and SS-B/La, may be especially harmful to the growing fetus and newborn. They attack heart tissue, skin, blood cells (white cells, red cells, and platelets), and the liver. The most serious of these problems is permanent, complete heart block, which may be life-threatening. In heart block, the normal electrical signal stimulating and regulating the fetal heartbeat is interrupted or damaged by the maternal autoantibodies or by other still unidentified associated factors. The result is an abnormally slow heart rate. The cardiac dysfunction usually becomes manifest between 20 and 30 weeks of gestation, most frequently at or about 24 weeks. This slow fetal heart rate can be identified by routine examination, obstetrical sonogram, or special fetal echocardiogram. In almost all cases, the heart block is an isolated problem; there are no structural deformities of the heart.

Curiously, the presence of these autoantibodies is not associated with heart problems in the mother, only in her offspring. In contrast to the heart, which is damaged during pregnancy, the skin rash is generally manifest only after birth, most commonly in the first to third months of life. Importantly, the skin rash can be triggered by sun exposure. It often involves the eyelids, face, and scalp. It is generally very red and can have a circular appearance. Liver abnormalities and low blood counts are rare problems but should be checked for. Like the rash, these abnormalities are not permanent. Most affected children have either heart block or skin rashes, but some have both. Studies suggest that girls are more often affected by the rash than boys, but both sexes are equally susceptible to heart block.

### Anti-SS-A/Ro and Anti-SS-B/La Antibodies

The harmful antibodies thus far identified by numerous investigators are directed against normal cellular components called Ro or SS-A and La or SS-B. The SS-A/Ro and SS-B/La proteins are thought to exist together in a single particle that is present in all cells. Therefore, it is difficult to explain why other fetal organs, as well as the mother's heart, are not damaged. SS-A/Ro is composed of two separate proteins of different sizes: 52 kilodaltons (kD) and 60 kD. La is one 48-kD protein. Antibodies to SS-A/Ro and SS-B/La occur in approximately 60–100 percent of patients with Sjogren's syndrome. They are less frequent in SLE. Antibodies to the 52SS-A/Ro protein are more common in individuals with Sjogren's syndrome than in those with SLE. With regard to neonatal lupus, it is not certain which antibody—anti-52SS-A/Ro, anti-60SS-A/Ro, or anti-48SS-B/La—is most important. All women with Sjogren's syndrome should be tested for these antibodies as part of prepregnancy counseling. If the antibodies are present, then special fetal cardiac monitoring can be performed during the pregnancy.

The methods of testing for these autoantibodies are important because tests differ in their sensitivity. Some tests are capable of detecting very small quantities of these antibodies. This is relevant because at present it is not certain whether it is solely the quantity of antibody or some still unknown quality of the antibody that is critical in causing fetal heart damage. The patient's serum (the clear liquid part of the blood that does not contain cells) is used for all testing. The least sensitive test, which may not detect lower titers of antibodies, is called immunodiffusion. Currently, the most widely used test, which is more sensitive than immunodiffusion, is the enzyme-linked immunoabsorbent assay (ELISA), in which a patient's serum is analyzed for antibodies against highly purified forms of SS-A/Ro and SS-B/La. Most ELISAs do not distinguish between the 52 and 60 forms of SS-A/Ro. A third test, the immunoblot or Western blot, is sensitive and can distinguish antibodies to the two different components of SS-A/Ro, although the test picks up the 52SS-A/Ro more effectively. The ELISA is available in commonly used commercial laboratories and most university medical centers. Immunoblot may be done only in certain specialized centers. If it is required, serum can be safely sent by normal mail delivery to such centers. In the author's experience, immunoblot may be helpful. Women who have anti-SS-A/Ro antibodies but who may be at lower risk for heart block than other women with anti-SS-A/Ro antibodies have three characteristics:

1  When their serum is tested by ELISA, they have only low titers of antibodies to SS-A/Ro.

2  By ELISA or immunoblot, they have no associated anti-SS-B/La antibodies.

3  By immunoblot, they do not have antibodies to the 52SS-A/Ro.

While heart block has never been associated with any other autoantibodies, the skin rash has rarely been linked with antibodies to another cellular protein called UI RNA-protein (UI RNP).

### The Risks

If a mother is found to have antibodies against SS-A/Ro and SS-B/La, what then is the risk of having a baby with cardiac, cutaneous, or hematological manifestations of neonatal lupus? There is some controversy regarding the exact percentages, but generally the chances are between 1 and 5 in 100 pregnancies if a mother has anti-SS-A/Ro or SS-B/La antibodies. Although this still appears to be a low risk, it is far higher than the reported incidence of heart block occurring in the general population. It is very puzzling that many women with these same antibodies have totally healthy children. These are areas of active investigation.

### Management of the Mother at Risk

What should be done to prevent a problem once the mother's risk is identified? The answer depends largely on whether this is a first pregnancy or whether heart block or any other manifestation of neonatal lupus has previously occurred in an offspring. In the first situation, a conservative approach is warranted. Management should consist of an echocardiogram sometime around the 18th week of pregnancy. This may be repeated at or about the 24th week and then again around 30 weeks. From this point on, routine obstetrical care (listening to the baby's heart rate) may be sufficient. Should a problem in the fetal heart be detected, therapies (described below) directed at lowering antibody levels or simply attempting to treat the heart condition may be justified. However, the situation is a bit of a "Catch 22" in that once established, heart block is not likely to be reversed. The outcome at this point ranges from death in utero to a normal life even without a pacemaker. Thus, the choice of management in a first pregnancy is difficult given the varying outcomes and the rarity of the disease.

In the mother with known antibodies who has already had a child with heart block, the risk of having a second affected child may be as high as one in six. In the author's series, there have only been 9 cases of recurrent heart block in 50 subsequent pregnancies in 50 mothers. It is possible to have one child with heart block and a second child with a rash or vice versa. Do these odds justify aggressive management in the early weeks of pregnancy? This is a very unsettled issue but again, given the fact that the majority of fetuses will not develop heart block, prophylactic therapies are not recommended. The use of procedures such as plasmapheresis and/or steroids prior to the detection of a problem is not justified at this time. The former procedure is time-consuming and requires up to three 3–6-hour sessions per week, during which time the patient has blood removed and cleansed of the antibody. It should be noted that there is no exchange with another person's blood. Perhaps the optimal management is a weekly echocardiogram between the 18th and 30th weeks of pregnancy (more frequently than is recommended for a mother who has never had a child with heart block). If the fetus is found to have heart block, there are circumstances in which therapy may be initiated. Most physicians advise just watching and performing weekly echocardiograms if third-degree (complete) heart block is present and there are no signs of heart failure. (In heart failure, the heart is not able to pump the blood adequately.) If the heartbeat indicated second-degree (incomplete) block, it is theoretically possible (but never proven) that treatment of the mother with a steroid such as dexamethasone, which can cross the placenta and enter the fetal circulation, will reverse the block before it becomes third-degree. Unfortunately, in almost all situations, the block is already complete at the time of first identification. If the fetus shows signs of inflammation such as fluid around the heart, lungs, or abdomen, this may be a more ominous sign and dexamethasone may be initiated. Clearly, more research is needed before definite recommendations can be made.

## Prognosis for the Baby with Neonatal Lupus

The long-term outlook for the child with heart block is generally good. However, the heart block is permanent, and in some cases the condition is fatal. In the author's experience, in 22 (19 percent) of 113 children, the majority of the deaths occurred when the infants were less than 3 months old. Most children do require pacemakers that are probably needed for life. In the author's experience with 113 children, 66 (58 percent) required pacemakers. In another study from Canada, 38 (57 percent) of 67 children required pacemakers. Pacemakers are often implanted in the first 3 months of life.

For the child with only skin manifestations of neonatal lupus, the prognosis is excellent. The rash generally disappears by about 8 months to 1 year of life. In most cases, no medications are needed and there are no scars or marks.

There is no evidence to suggest that children with neonatal lupus will eventually develop SLE in later life. However, any child born to a mother with SLE does have a higher risk of developing lupus later on, especially if the child is a girl. The chances are probably no more than 1 in 10.

In summary, the presence of antibodies to SS-A/Ro and SS-B/La poses a risk, albeit small, to the developing fetus. Currently, numerous laboratories are investigating the mechanisms of this problem in an attempt to identify high-risk pregnancies more specifically and to develop treatment plans that might prevent heart block from occurring. To accomplish this important task, a national research registry for neonatal lupus has been established at the Hospital for Joint Diseases in New York City through funding by the National Institute of Arthritis, Musculoskeletal, and Skin Diseases. It is hoped that all mothers with affected children will enroll in this important Registry.

## Other Problems Facing the Prospective Mother with Sjogren's Syndrome

Some individuals with Sjogren's syndrome have antiphospholipid antibodies (see Chapter 19) called anticardiolipin antibodies. These can be tested for by ELISA. The so-called lupus anticoagulant is another type of antiphospholipid antibody and can be tested for by special clotting tests such as partial thromboplastin time (PTT) or dilute Russell viper venom time (dRVVT). These antibodies are important because they are associated with recurrent miscarriages, most often in the second trimester. Research suggests that these antibodies may cause clots to form in the placenta and thereby interrupt blood flow to the fetus. Various treatments are available to prevent fetal loss, including aspirin, heparin, and prednisone. Each regimen carries a risk, and therapies must be individualized.

**Elise Belilos, MD**

**Steven Carsons, MD**

# 19 The Antiphospholipid Antibody Syndrome

LIKE SJOGREN'S SYNDROME, the antiphospholipid antibody syndrome is an autoimmune disorder marked by the production of autoantibodies. In this syndrome, the presence of these autoantibodies is associated with an increased risk of clotting events. Also like Sjogren's syndrome, the antiphospholipid antibody syndrome can occur as a primary disorder or in association with connective tissue diseases such as systemic lupus erythematosus, rheumatoid arthritis, or Sjogren's syndrome.

In the medical literature, several different names for this syndrome have been used, such as the lupus anticoagulant syndrome, the anticardiolipin antibody syndrome, and the antiphospholipid antibody syndrome. Historically, it was originally called the lupus anticoagulant syndrome, as it was first described in patients with systemic lupus erythematosus and because the laboratory findings mimic those of an anticoagulant (blood-thinning) effect. However, it was soon realized that not only did it occur in patients without lupus, but that patients with this syndrome actually had a tendency to develop thrombotic (clotting) disorders. Later, specific antibodies directed against cardiolipin (a fatty material derived from beef heart) were described, and the syndrome was then referred to as the anticardiolipin antibody syndrome. However, since cardiolipin is included in a broader biochemical group known as phospholipids, the more general term antiphospholipid antibody syndrome is currently preferred.

## Clinical Findings

The clinical syndrome is characterized by recurrent clotting in the arteries and/or veins. Common manifestations include deep vein thrombosis (phlebitis), usually affecting the lower extremities. Patients may note swelling and pain in the leg, and the extremity may appear warm and red. When a physician suspects phlebitis, he or she will usually order a Doppler study of the involved area. This test can demonstrate clotting in the affected veins. It is important to diagnose and treat deep vein phlebitis promptly, as clots in the leg may travel to the lungs (pulmonary embolus). In addition to clots in the veins, patients may have clots in the arteries that may lead to coronary thrombosis (heart attack) or neurological symptoms. Neurological involvement commonly includes stroke or transient ischemic attack (TIA or mini-stroke). These may present as permanent or transient loss of vision, slurred speech, or weakness and/or numbness of an extremity. Patients may also have cardiac valvular problems (sterile endocarditis, Libman-Sacks endocarditis) and consequently may need to take antibiotic prophylaxis for dental or other invasive procedures. Women with the antiphospholipid antibody syndrome may have recurrent spontaneous miscarriages. These are often late miscarriages, occurring in the second and third trimesters, and are believed to be primarily on the basis of placental thrombosis. Patients with the antiphospholipid antibody syndrome may also have a rash known as livedo reticularis that appears as a lacy, mottled pattern, most commonly seen on the extremities.

## Diagnostic Testing

When a physician suspects the antiphospholipid antibody syndrome, several different laboratory tests should be ordered to confirm the diagnosis. Patients often have low platelet counts (thrombocytopenia). The partial thromboplastin time (PTT) may be elevated; this is one of a series of clotting assays that can be used to detect a "circulating anticoagulant." In addition, specific anticardiolipin antibodies can be measured. Patients may also have a false-positive VDRL test for syphilis (a positive blood test in the absence of syphilis infection) due to the fact that the antibodies used to detect syphilis infection are also directed against phospholipids. An individual patient with the antiphospholipid antibody syndrome may have abnormalities in one or any combination of these tests.

Thus, to adequately evaluate a patient for this syndrome, it is necessary to obtain a series of laboratory tests.

## Association of the Antiphospholipid Antibody Syndrome with Other Autoimmune Disorders

It is not unusual for multiple autoimmune disorders to occur in one individual. This is best demonstrated by secondary Sjogren's syndrome, which, by definition, occurs in individuals who have another autoimmune connective tissue disease such as rheumatoid arthritis or systemic lupus erythematosus. Similarly, the secondary antiphospholipid antibody syndrome may occur in individuals who have an established autoimmune connective tissue disease. Most commonly, the secondary antiphospholipid antibody syndrome occurs in patients with systemic lupus erythematosus. However, it has also been reported to occur in patients with other connective tissue diseases including Sjogren's syndrome. Patients with the antiphospholipid antibody syndrome associated with Sjogren's syndrome may have a lower incidence of clotting problems than do patients with the primary antiphospholipid syndrome or lupus-associated antiphospholipid antibody syndrome. Nonetheless, Sjogren's syndrome patients who develop thromboses at a young age should be suspected of having the antiphospholipid antibody syndrome. Similarly, if a woman with Sjogren's syndrome has multiple miscarriages, she should be tested for antiphospholipid and related antibodies. When a woman possesses both antiphospholipid and SS-A/SS-B (see Chapter 18), fetal loss due to placental clotting (antiphospholipid antibody syndrome) should be differentiated from fetal loss due to congenital heart block (SS-A/SS-B).

## Treatment and Prophylaxis

Since the antiphospholipid antibody syndrome is associated with multiple clotting events, treatment is primarily with anticoagulants (blood thinners). Patients with the syndrome who have had recurrent major thrombotic events (such as deep vein thrombosis, pulmonary embolus, or stroke) generally require lifelong anticoagulation with warfarin (Coumadin). Patients with relatively minor or not clearly documented thrombotic events may be treated with aspirin alone. Patients who have positive blood tests but have not had any clinical manifestations of the antiphospholipid antibody syndrome or thrombotic events do not necessarily have to be treated. In women with the antiphospholipid antibody syndrome who have had recurrent spontaneous miscarriages, a combination of aspirin and subcutaneous heparin injections has been used during pregnancy in an attempt to maintain the pregnancy. Coumadin is known to be teratogenic (causes birth defects) and should never be taken by women who plan to become pregnant.

In summary, the manifestations of the antiphospholipid antibody syndrome and the circumstances (e.g., a desire for pregnancy) can vary greatly from patient to patient. Thus, the treatment for the antiphospholipid antibody syndrome should be individualized.

# Treatment
## and Management

Gary Rosenblum, DO

Steven Carsons, MD

# 20 Treatment of Systemic Manifestations of Sjogren's Syndrome

WHILE MOST PERSONS with Sjogren's syndrome require only local moisturizing therapy for their symptoms of xerostomia (dry mouth) or keratoconjunctivitis sicca (KCS, dry eyes), occasionally systemic medication is necessary for extraglandular involvement. The scope of extraglandular involvement is covered in Chapters 9–16. Additionally, persons with secondary Sjogren's syndrome often require medication for their primary condition (usually a connective tissue disease; see Chapter 8). Nonsteroidal anti-inflammatory drugs, corticosteroids, and immunomodulating drugs comprise the major groups of systemic medication used in Sjogren's syndrome. The choice of therapy depends on the individual's specific case. A risk benefit analysis is necessary for every physician and patient before initiating medication. This chapter will review the general indications, common side effects, and guidelines for safe use of systemic therapy.

## Nonsteroidal Anti-inflammatory Drugs

Nonsteroidal anti-inflammatory drugs (NSAIDs) are widely used in the treatment of connective tissue and rheumatic diseases. In addition to prescription NSAIDs, a number of over-the-counter (OTC) NSAIDs are available and frequently used by the public. Over 100 million prescriptions are written for NSAIDs per year. NSAIDs are derivatives of aspirin and have properties similar to those of aspirin. Depending on the person'ssize, concomitant drug use, and other physiological factors, 12 to 24 aspirin tablets would have to be consumed daily to equal the anti-inflammatory effect of a full-dose NSAID. Therefore, NSAIDs are usually better tolerated than aspirin.

NSAIDs and aspirin suppress inflammation and reduce pain through their effects on inflammatory mediators (primarily prostaglandins). Specifically, they inhibit cyclooxygenase, an enzyme responsible for the production of prostaglandins. Although cyclooxygenase and prostaglandins are found in inflammatory cells, they are expressed in other tissues that depend on their presence for normal function. Cyclooxygenase inhibition may cause side effects in tissues such as the stomach and kidneys. Newer NSAIDs that target cyclooxygenase in inflammatory cells have recently been marketed.

Sjogren's syndrome patients are most commonly prescribed NSAIDs for joint pains, muscle aches, and constitutional features (usually fever and fatigue). Occasionally, NSAIDs are used for the discomfort of glandular swelling. However, little improvement in salivary or lacrimal (tear) flow rates has been noted, and the course of glandular inflammation and swelling is not altered. While NSAIDs may help the discomfort of glandular swelling, they do not prevent or cure xerostomia or KCS.

NSAID-induced side effects are fairly frequent, although usually mild. Gastrointestinal (GI) complaints are the most common adverse effects, especially abdominal discomfort and diarrhea. More severe though less common effects include peptic ulcer formation (gastric ulcers more commonly than duodenal ulcers), gastritis, esophagitis, and bleeding. A prior history of peptic ulcer disease and concurrent use of corticosteroids may increase the GI side effects. Strategies to minimize GI side effects include taking NSAIDs with food, avoiding other NSAIDs or aspirin products (unless specifically prescribed), and using prescription antacid and cytoprotective medications. Misoprostol is a fairly new medication that may prevent gastric ulcer formation in persons taking NSAIDs. Its use is suggested in patients at high risk for ulcers, including the elderly and those with prior peptic ulcer disease. H2 blockers are the major group of prescription antacid medications. These drugs may reduce GI side effects and limit the formation of duodenal ulcers; however, unlike misoprostol, they are not currently approved for ulcer prevention. Many of the H2 blockers, such as Pepcid AC, are now available without a prescription.

Other potential side effects of aspirin and NSAIDs include elevation of blood pressure, fluid retention with swelling around the feet and ankles, elevation of liver enzymes, changes in kidney function, and easy bruising and bleeding (due to a mild blood-thinning effect). These effects are usually reversible upon discontinuation of the NSAID. Persons with known liver or kidney disease and those with bleeding disorders or presently taking a blood thinner should consult their physician before using NSAIDs (whether prescription or OTC). NSAIDs and aspirin should be discontinued approximately 10 days before any dental or surgical procedure to diminish the risk of enhanced bleeding.

Over 20 NSAIDs are marketed in the United States. There are distinct differences in the pharmacokinetics (body utilization) of NSAIDs, although these differences do not make one NSAID superior to another. Physicians must individualize their choice of NSAID therapy based on the patient's past medical history, coexisting medications, and compliance with the medication regimen. Table 9 lists the most common NSAIDs, their recommended daily dose, and the frequency of dosing.

### Corticosteroids

Corticosteroids are powerful suppressors of inflammation used in certain arthritic and rheumatic conditions. When first introduced (about 1950) as a treatment for arthritis, they were thought to be miracle drugs. However, their tremendous early benefits were followed by adverse effects in some individuals, leading to great caution in their use. Corticosteroids reduce inflammation by interacting with different cells and components of the immune system. Examples of corticosteroids include prednisone, cortisone, methylprednisolone, and dexamethasone.

Physicians most commonly prescribe corticosteroids in tablet or capsule form. Other methods exist, depending on the particular problem. In patients who cannot take medicine orally, corticosteroids can be injected into the muscle (intramuscular) or vein (intravenous) and still work throughout the body. In certain serious situations, high-dose corticosteroids are given intravenously in multiple doses, known as pulse therapy. Corticosteroids can be injected into a local area of inflammation, such as in tendonitis or bursitis. Arthritis limited to one joint may be treated by an intra-articular (into the joint) injection. Rashes may be treated with topical corticosteroid creams or lotions.

All corticosteroids are related to cortisol, a naturally occurring hormone that controls and affects numerous body functions. Cortisol and other hormones are produced in the adrenal glands. When used for most

**TABLE 9   THE MOST COMMON NSAIDS**

| Drug (Brand Name) | Available Strengths (mg) | Frequency of Dose(s) |
|---|---|---|
| Choline magnesium trisalicylate (Trilisate) | 500, 750, 1,000 | 2 × day |
| Diclofenac potassium (Cataflam) | 50 | 3 × day |
| Diclofenac sodium (Voltaren) (Voltaren XR) | 25, 50, 75<br>100 (XR) | 2 × day<br>1 × day |
| Diflunisal (Dolobid) | 250, 500 | 2 × day |
| Etodolac (Lodine) (Lodine XL) | 200, 300, 400, 500<br>400, 600 | 2–4 × day<br>1–2 × day |
| Flurbiprofen (Ansaid) | 50, 100 | 2–3 × day |
| Ibuprofen (Motrin, Advil) | 200, 400, 600, 800 | 3 × day |
| Indomethacin (Indocin) (Indocin SR) | 25, 50<br>75 (SR) | 2–3 × day<br>1 × day |
| Ketoprofen (Orudis) (Oruvail) | 25, 50, 75<br>100, 150, 200 | 2–3 × day<br>1 × day |
| Ketorolac tromethamine (Toradol) | 10 | 2 × day* |
| Nabumetone (Relafen) | 500, 750 | 1–2 × day |
| Naproxen (Naprosyn) | 375, 500 | 2 × day |
| Naproxen sodium (Anaprox) (Naprelan) | 275, 550<br>375, 500 | 2–3 × day<br>1–2 × day |
| Oxaprozin (Daypro) | 600 | 1–2 × day |
| Piroxicam (Feldene) | 10, 20 | 1 × day |
| Salsalate (Disalcid) (Mono-Gesic) Salflex) | 500, 750<br>750<br>500, 750 | 2–3 × day |
| Sulindac (Clinoril) | 150, 200 | 2 × day |
| Tolmentin sodium (Tolectin) | 200, 400, 600 | 3–4 × day |

* Not for prolonged use

medical conditions, corticosteroids are given in doses that exceed the amount of cortisol made in the adrenals. At these doses, the adrenal glands are suppressed and their cortisol production is reduced. With prolonged intake of corticosteroids, the adrenal glands slowly shrink. Since cortisol is necessary for numerous body functions, corticosteroids cannot be discontinued abruptly; they must be reduced slowly to allow the adrenal glands to regain their function and produce enough cortisol. Therefore, steroid dose changes should be directed by a physician.

Corticosteroids have no role in the glandular disease of Sjogren's syndrome. In the rare patient who has internal organ involvement, such as that of the lung, kidney, or nervous system, corticosteroids may be prescribed. Additionally, patients who develop vasculitis (inflammation of the blood vessels and resultant damage to the organs supplied by those vessels) are often placed on corticosteroids. Patients requiring corticosteroids are often very ill and are usually hospitalized at some point in the course of their disease. Occasionally, inflammatory arthritis occurs in a Sjogren's syndrome patient who is otherwise not ill; this may require the use of a corticosteroid. Persons with secondary Sjogren's syndrome and underlying connective tissue disease usually take corticosteroids for their primary disease. This is especially true for people with systemic lupus erythematosus and rheumatoid arthritis.

## Side Effects of Corticosteroids

Corticosteroids can make a tremendous difference in the outcome of some Sjogren's syndrome patients and may even be a lifesaving treatment. However, they have numerous potential side effects, most of which are infrequent. These side effects are somewhat dependent on the amount and duration of use. Frequent side effects include increased appetite and weight gain, increased risk of osteoporosis, impaired wound healing, increased risk of infection, and risk of abnormal growth in children. Less common side effects include muscle weakness, bone pain and damage (osteonecrosis), high blood pressure, thin fragile skin, elevated cholesterol, fluid retention and swelling, diabetes mellitus, cataracts, and psychiatric symptoms. Uncommon and rare side effects include peptic ulcer disease, glaucoma, electrolyte disturbance, pancreatitis, increased hair growth, impotence, and secondary amenorrhea.

Regarding these side effects, persons with any of the aforementioned conditions need special consideration and strategies to prevent worsening of their disorders before using corticosteroids. Osteoporosis and fracture prevention should be discussed with all patients taking corticosteroids. Proper calcium and vitamin D intake is important, as well as a well-balanced diet. Regular weight-bearing exercise such as walking is helpful in the treatment of osteoporosis. Other lifestyle changes may be helpful, such as avoiding smoking and excessive alcohol intake. Strategies to prevent falls, such as guardrails and bathing chairs, are very helpful, especially in elderly patients. Estrogen therapy (or hormonal replacement therapy [HRT]) is still considered an optimal treatment for certain women at risk for osteoporosis, whether steroid or nonsteroid induced. For those who cannot take HRT, two recently approved drugs (alendronate and calcitonin nasal spray) may be considered for the treatment of osteoporosis. These are generally well tolerated, with minimal side effects. Patients with systemic lupus erythematosus or other rheumatic conditions are often discouraged from taking estrogen and may be candidates for these newer medications for osteoporosis.

Persons with high blood pressure should continue taking their medications while taking corticosteroids. Occasionally, physicians may need to increase the dose. Proper diet and avoidance of salt are prudent as well. Diabetics need close monitoring of their blood sugar while taking corticosteroids. Insulin and oral diabetic medications may have to be adjusted. Low-cholosterol diets should be encouraged, and monitoring of cholesterol blood levels should be maintained; if necessary, the physician may prescribe a cholesterol-lowering agent.

Since the risk of infection is increased while taking corticosteroids, persistent high fevers associated with shakes or chills warrant a call to the physician. Routine care with the primary care physician and ophthalmologist is recommended.

### Immunomodulating Agents

Immunomodulating agents are medications that have various immune functions and different methods of suppressing inflammation. They are often used in rheumatic conditions as adjunctive therapy to NSAIDs or corticosteroids. These medications begin to act very slowly, taking anywhere from 4 weeks to 4 months; therefore, they are not used for acute pain relief. Immunomodulating agents are intended to "turn off" the underlying inflammatory process in many rheumatic disorders and thus induce a remission. Additionally, by controlling the disease process, these agents hopefully permit the reduction of corticosteroids and even allow some patients to discontinue taking them. Examples of immunomodulating agents are hydroxychloroquine, methotrexate, azathioprine, cyclophosphamide, and gold compounds.

At this time, our understanding of the role of immunomodulating agents in Sjogren's syndrome is limited. As with corticosteroids, they are generally used in patients who have internal organ (usually lung, kidney, or nerve) involvement or vasculitis.

Hydroxychloroquine, a milder immunomodulating drug, is occasionally used for glandular involvement in Sjogren's syndrome patients and will be discussed further below. The remaining agents are used only for more serious complications or internal organ involvement. Studies have not shown these medications to relieve the symptoms or outcome of glandular disease (xerostomia and KCS).

## Hydroxychloroquine

Hydroxychloroquine is an antimalarial drug that has been used for decades in rheumatoid arthritis. The use of this drug in other rheumatic conditions continues to expand, including systemic lupus erythematosus, juvenile arthritis, and Sjogren's syndrome. The anti-inflammatory effect of hydroxychloroquine helps to relieve swelling, stiffness, and pain in patients with arthritis. Some systemic lupus erythematosus patients appear to sustain control or remission of their disease with hydroxychloroquine. It is particularly helpful for skin rashes and constitutional (fatigue and fever) features in lupus patients. These effects have been noted in Sjogren's syndrome patients as well. Studies have shown improvement in numerous laboratory abnormalities in Sjogren's syndrome patients, which may reduce the development of complications. However, no definitive improvement in glandular symptoms or decrease in glandular destruction has been demonstrated.

Hydroxychloroquine is available in tablet form and is usually very well tolerated. Potential side effects include diarrhea, loss of appetite, nausea and vomiting, headaches, upset stomach, and skin rash. Rarely, hydroxychloroquine can cause deposits in the cornea or retina of the eye. For this reason, eye exams by an ophthalmologist are required before initiating therapy and routinely (approximately every 4–6 months) while taking hydroxychloroquine. These deposits are usually unnoticed by patients and are most often reversible upon discontinuation of the medication. If persistent visual symptoms develop while taking hydroxy-chloroquine, a visit to the ophthalmologist is recommended.

## Methotrexate

Methotrexate is a folic acid (a vitamin B) inhibitor that interferes with cell growth. It acts as an anti-inflammatory and immunomodulating agent. It is used very often in rheumatoid arthritis patients and is believed to be extremely effective. Originally designed as a cancer therapy, it is now used in patients with multiple rheumatic conditions and other inflammatory disorders. The most common use of methotrexate in Sjogren's syndrome is in secondary disease when rheumatoid arthritis is the primary condition. Occasionally, patients with primary Sjogren's syndrome who have extraglandular internal organ involvement will be given methotrexate. While studies of methotrexate for glandular disease are pending, it is often used in rheumatic disease in the hope of lessening or discontinuing corticosteroids (steroid-sparing effect).

Methotrexate is available in tablet and intramuscular form. It is generally taken only 1 day per week. During treatment, doses are often split during that day. Generally, methotrexate is well tolerated. At low doses, mild side effects include upset stomach with nausea and vomiting, loss of appetite, diarrhea, and mouth sores. Another potential side effect is a decrease in blood cell counts that can increase the risk of infection or bleeding, depending on the cell type involved. Additionally, anemia can develop and cause weakness or fatigue. Because methotrexate can cause lung damage in rare instances, any history of prior lung disease should be reviewed with a physician prior to starting methotrexate. Patients taking methotrexate who develop a cough or progressive shortness of breath need immediate evaluation by their physician. In rare instances, liver problems may develop. Alcohol may increase the risk of liver disease and is prohibited with the use of methotrexate. Persons with a history of hepatitis infection need further evaluation before methotrexate therapy is considered. Due to the above possible side effects, frequent monitoring of patients on methotrexate is necessary. Routine examination and blood work (approximately every 4–6 weeks) are suggested to detect the development of any problem as early as possible.

## Cyclophosphamide

Cyclophosphamide is a very potent medication that affects cellular function and demonstrates a marked anti-inflammatory effect. Similar to methotrexate, its role in Sjogren's syndrome is reserved for seriously ill patients with internal organ involvement and/or vasculitis. In rare instances, it is used as a steroid-sparing agent. Cyclophosphamide may be used as part of a chemotherapy regimen in Sjogren's syndrome patients who develop lymphoma or pseudolymphoma.

Although this drug can be lifesaving, the side effects are substantial and limit its use. Common side effects include upset stomach with nausea and vomiting, hair loss, increased risk of infection, and decreased blood cell counts that can lead to bleeding or anemia. Other side effects include bladder abnormalities, such as bleeding and an increased risk of developing bladder cancer. Reproductive organ dysfunction, occasionally severe enough to lead to ovarian or testicular failure, can occur. This is dependent on the amount of cyclophosphamide received, as well as on the age of the patient. There may be an increased risk for the development of leukemias or lymphomas with cyclophosphamide. Because cyclophosphamide is harmful to the fetus, it is contraindicated during pregnancy.

The use of immunomodulating agents is confined to a very few individuals with Sjogren's syndrome. The physician will consider the potential risks and benefits of the medications in every case. Close monitoring by the physician and patient is crucial for the best outcome while using these agents.

**Troy E. Daniels, DDS, MS**
**Ernest Newbrun, DMD, PhD**

# 21  Oral Treatment and Prevention of Tooth Decay

THESE CLINICAL GUIDELINES are primarily for healthcare professionals providing oral treatment and prevention of tooth decay for their patients with Sjogren's syndrome. They are also for Sjogren's syndrome patients to help them better understand the often complex treatment that may be necessary. Some of the included drugs or materials require a prescription, and some of the procedures can be performed only by dentists.

## Dental Caries (Tooth Decay) Prevention and Treatment (for All Patients with Natural Teeth)
### Diet
Each patient must learn the role of dietary sugars in the development of tooth decay, as well as the need to limit sugar intake to meals and to eliminate it between meals. Foods, beverages, gum, and other products that contain noncariogenic sweetening agents (e.g., aspartame, sorbitol, saccharin, or xylitol) should be used whenever possible.

### Oral Hygiene
Each patient must learn how to remove dental plaque effectively, including the use of dental plaque staining and the correct use of a toothbrush and dental floss. Twice-daily tooth brushing with a fluoride-containing toothpaste (0.1 or 0.15 percent fluoride) and daily use of dental floss between all teeth are necessary. For some patients, electric

toothbrushes, irrigators, or supplementary oral hygiene aids may be recommended.

## Risk of Tooth Decay

The risk of tooth decay in an individual patient can be estimated from the severity of oral clinical signs (e.g., amount of clinically apparent saliva, mucosal stickiness, dental decalcification), measurement of saliva production, and estimation of caries-producing organisms in the saliva:

- Clinical signs of hyposalivation (less than normal) include the presence of new or recurrent decay on the root surface or incisal edge, sticky mucosal surfaces, absence of expressible saliva from the major salivary ducts, and absence of pooled saliva in the mouth floor.

- Measure stimulated whole salivary flow (in millimeters per minute) by asking the patient to chew paraffin wax (1 g) for 5 minutes and collect the saliva in a graduated tube. If flow is <0.5 ml/min (or <0.5 mg/ml), the patient is at much higher than normal risk of developing tooth decay.

- Kits suitable for the culture and estimation of *Streptococcus mutans* are commercially available. If the amount of salivary *S. mutans* exceeds $1 \times 10^6$ colony forming units per milliliter of whole saliva, a 1-minute twice-daily rinse with 0.12 percent chlorhexidine (Peridex or PerioGard) for 2 weeks should be prescribed.

## Topical Fluoride

Topical fluoride can be professionally applied and self-applied:

- At a dental office, a high-concentration agent can be applied, such as 1.23 percent acidulated phosphate fluoride gel (many brands are available) for 4 minutes in a tray or 2.25 percent fluoride varnish (Duraflor) directly onto the teeth. These applications can be repeated every 6 months or more frequently if necessary.

- Self-applied fluorides must be specifically prescribed and their application demonstrated to the patient. The methods to be used depend on the severity of the tooth decay and/or the degree of salivary hypofunction.

- Patients at low to moderate risk of tooth decay should use a 0.05 percent sodium fluoride rinse for 1–2 minutes at least once daily before going to sleep.

- Patients at high risk of tooth decay should apply 1.1 percent neutral sodium fluoride gel daily in custom-made trays for 5–10 minutes. They should then floss between all teeth immediately after tray removal to carry fluoride to those adjoining dental surfaces. This is best done just before going to sleep.

### Dental Restoration

In restoring decayed teeth, conservative preparations should be used. Light-cured glass ionomer cements should be used where practical because they release fluoride and are more resistant to marginal decay. *Note*: For initial treatment of these patients, dental restorations with subgingival margins (those that end under the gum) should be avoided wherever possible. This is because subgingival margins are less accessible to topical fluoride, they are the usual site of recurrent decay, and decay there is more difficult to detect and treat. Full-veneer crowns, if ultimately necessary, should *not* be placed until caries are under complete control (i.e., the patient has been free of new cavities for at least 1 year).

### Recall Examinations

At each recall visit, visual examination of dental surfaces should be supplemented with bite wing radiographs (X-ray images of the visible parts of the back teeth) as needed, and the oral mucosa should be examined for signs of candidiasis (infection with *Candida*). The patient's dental plaque control should be reassessed by use of a plaque stain and plaque control techniques should be reinforced. The amount of salivary *S. mutans* can be monitored and a chlorhexidine rinse prescribed again as needed.

### Oral Candidiasis: Diagnosis and Treatment
### Diagnosis

About one-third of patients with chronic hyposalivation develop oral candidiasis, usually of the erythematous (red) type. Adequate treatment usually provides significant improvement of oral symptoms in spite of continuing oral dryness.

TABLE 10   TOPICAL ANTIFUNGAL DRUGS FOR TREATING ORAL CANDIDIASIS IN
PATIENTS WITH LITTLE SALIVA

| Drug and Form | Dose[†] | Comments |
|---|---|---|
| Nystatin vaginal tablets 100,000 U/tablet | 2–4/day | Dissolve each tablet slowly (15 minutes) in the mouth, using sips of water as necessary to aid dissolution; has a medicinal taste; contains lactose |
| Clotrimazole vaginal tablets 100 mg/tablet | ½ tablet b.i.d. | Dissolve slowly in the mouth, as for nystatin vaginal tablets; use if there has been an inadequate response to nystatin |
| Nystatin creme 100,000 U/g | 2–3 times/day | For treating angular cheilitis; usually used concurrently with an antifungal drug taken by mouth |
| Nystatin topical powder 100,000 U/g | 2 times/day | Apply a fairly even coating to the fitting surface of a clean, moistened denture; this supplements other antifungal drugs taken by mouth and may be helpful in maintenance therapy |

* These drugs have little or no risk of supporting dental caries with prolonged use in patients with significant salivary hypofunction. All are unflavored.

† The treatment period for erythematous candidiasis in patients with salivary hypofunction ranges from about 4 weeks to several months, but pseudomembranous oral candidiasis usually requires only 1–2 weeks of treatment.

Symptoms of oral candidiasis include a burning sensation of the mucosa, intolerance of acidic or spicy foods, and a change in taste or development of a metallic taste.

Candidiasis is recognized by its clinical signs: erythema (redness) on the dorsal tongue, palate, buccal mucosa, or denture-bearing mucosa, atrophy of the filiform papillae on the dorsal tongue, and angular cheilitis (sores at the corners of the mouth). The diagnosis is confirmed by fungal culture of a swab specimen from such a mucosal lesion, which reveals significant numbers of colony-forming units of a *Candida* species.

## Treatment

Treating oral candidiasis in patients with chronic salivary hypofunction usually requires the use of topical forms of polyene or imidazole antifungal drugs that *do not contain* sucrose or glucose for periods of weeks or months (Table 10). Topical forms are needed because systemically administered drugs do not reach the mouths of patients with severe hyposalivation in therapeutically adequate amounts. The drug used must not increase the patient's risk of developing dental caries. Unfortunately, all the topical oral forms of antifungal drugs currently available contain large amounts of glucose or sucrose, which often lead to tooth decay.

Generally, the best topical antifungal drug for use in patients who have remaining natural teeth is nystatin vaginal tablets (which contain lactose but not sucrose or glucose). They must be dissolved slowly in the mouth for 15–20 minutes two or three times a day. If the patient's mouth is very dry, frequent sips of water may be necessary to allow the tablet to dissolve in that time.

For patients who wear partial or complete dentures, additional instructions and treatment are needed: (1) Dentures must be removed from the mouth before the antifungal drug is applied. (2) Dentures must be disinfected by soaking them overnight in a substance compatible with the denture material (e.g., 1 percent sodium hypochlorite for dentures without exposed metal or benzalkonium chloride diluted 1:750 in water for dentures with exposed metal) and rinsed before reinserting them in the mouth. (3) Nystatin topical powder may be applied on the fitting surface of the denture when it is reinserted in the mouth.

The above treatments should be continued until the clinician has observed the healing of all oral erythematous (red) lesions, return of filiform papillae on the dorsal tongue, and disappearance of associated symptoms.

The presence of angular cheilitis almost always indicates concurrent candidiasis in the mouth. Angular cheilitis can be treated by nystatin or clotrimazole creme, but in most cases this substance should not be used without concurrently treating the intraoral infection.

After treatment is completed, recurrence is fairly common and the patient must be retreated as described above. If recurrence is frequent, retreatment should be immediately followed by maintenance therapy (e.g., continued use of half of a nystatin vaginal tablet slowly dissolved in the mouth each day).

### Salivary Flow Stimulation

The following methods of stimulating salivary flow are effective, but only in those patients who retain some salivary function.

## Physiological Stimulation

- *Sugarless* chewing gum (e.g., xylitol gum) or *sugarless* hard candies can be used as needed during the day to relieve oral symptoms.

- Either substance can increase salivary flow, but only while the gum or candy is present in the mouth.

## Pharmacological Stimulation

- Pilocarpine tablets (Salagen) can increase salivary flow for 1–2 hours after absorption by the body. This drug should not be used by patients who have a history of uncontrolled asthma, gastrointestinal ulcer, acute iritis or narrow-angle glaucoma, or by those who are pregnant. It may not be suitable for patients with unstable cardiovascular disease. Individual doses can be titrated, usually in the range between 5 mg three times per day and 10 mg four times per day.

### Use of Saliva Substitutes

Generally, these are helpful only for patients with fairly severe, continuous salivary hypofunction, particularly those wearing a complete denture. There are several types of saliva substitutes:

- Carboxymethylcellulose (CMC) based: Glandosane (without preservative), Moi-Stir, Orex, Salivart (without preservative), Xero-Lube (with fluoride and xylitol)
- CMC based with mucopolysaccharide: MouthKote (contains xylitol)
- Glycerate polymer based: Oral balance (contains xylitol)
- Mucin based: Orthana (not available in the United States)

Saliva substitutes are usually most helpful when used at the bedside, while talking, or while traveling. None replace all the functions of natural saliva, and none last long because they are swallowed. Some CMC-based products have lubrication and wetting properties that may be no better than those of water. The gel-based and mucopolysaccharide-containing products may last somewhat longer.

## Current Prescription Drug Use

The patient's current prescription drug use should be reviewed regularly to identify any drugs that decrease salivary function. If such a drug is being used, the problem should be discussed with the prescriber; it may be possible to eliminate the drug or to substitute one that has less effect on salivary function.

## Excessive Water Consumption

Patients should understand that dry mouth is seldom associated with systemic dehydration and that drinking large amounts of water does not overcome mouth dryness. Frequent small sips of water during the day help reduce oral symptoms. However, overuse of water will remove any mucus on the lining of the mouth and further increase the symptoms of dryness.

Patients may have frequent sleep interruption caused by nocturia from excessive water consumption at night. To avoid nocturia, patients should not drink water beginning 1 hour before sleep. Instead, a saliva substitute should be used.

*Note:* The authors do not endorse any product mentioned in these guidelines. Brand names of products are used when a generic description would be inadequate or when branded products are the only ones available.

# 22 Care of the Mouth, Throat, and Voice

THE VOICE IS AN INTEGRAL PART of our lives, yet we do not fully appreciate our voices until we either cannot speak comfortably or cannot speak at all. The lack of saliva in Sjogren's syndrome patients, with resulting dry mouth, may cause voice problems. Dry vocal cords do not always meet properly. When the Sjogren's syndrome patient then tries to "push out" the voice by forcing or attempting a pitch change, hoarseness occurs. The patient may also clear the throat frequently, causing excessive pressure on the vocal cords. Redness and edema (fluid accumulation) can further damage the cords.

### How Is the Voice Produced Normally?

The vocal cords act as a sound source to produce voice. During inhalation the air goes through the nose and mouth into the larynx, causing the vocal cords to part. The air then continues down the respiratory mechanism until it reaches the lungs. During exhalation the process is reversed, and as the air travels upward and reaches the larynx, the movement brings the cords together. Any alteration in mass, elasticity, or compliance can cause a voice problem.

### What Are Voice Disorders?

A voice disorder can be broadly defined as something that interferes with smooth, effortless sound. Voice problems are divided into the following categories:

1  Pitch: too high or low, falsetto, diplophonia (production of double tones)

2  Intensity: too loud or soft

3  Resonance: nasal or denasal

4  Quality

  a  Harsh or raspy

  b  Breathy—bowed vocal cords do not close completely, and air escapes

  c  Hoarse—combination of harsh and breathy

Subjective descriptions like these are instantaneous reactions to what the listener hears. In recent years, voice laboratories have provided more objective acoustic measurements of the voice.

### Organic and Functional Voice Disorders

Although voice disorders fall into two categories, organic (physical causes such as neurodegenerative diseases: multiple sclerosis or Parkinsons; maligned or paralyzed vocal fold lesions; and benign growths such as polyps and nodules) and functional (emotional and/or behavioral causes), the two can interact. For example, vocal abuse can lead to benign growths on the cords, which then makes the problem a physical or an organic disorder. The physical disorder can be cured, but a residual voice problem may remain.

### Types of Organic Voice Problems

1  Tumors are growths on the vocal cords that may be cancerous or benign. Nodules, polyps, and contact ulcers are always benign.

2  Papillomas are tumors caused by viruses and are associated with warts or herpes virus infection.

3  Paralyzed vocal cords can occur as a result of surgery, viral infection, or injury. Recovery is sometimes spontaneous.

4   Systemic problems with the voice may result from a generalized disease such as Sjogren's syndrome, which attacks different parts of the body. In Sjogren's syndrome, a dry larynx may become swollen and fatigued, so that when the patient coughs or clears the throat, the vocal cords are irritated.

5   Neurological diseases can cause vocal damage.

6   Respiratory disorders can cause vocal damage.

## Types of Functional Voice Problems

1   Emotional trauma

2   Personality problems

3   Vocal abuse/misuse such as habitual yelling, smoking, and excessive drinking

### Voice Therapy

Voice therapy helps to maximize the voice by teaching strategies for more effective vocal production. A trained listener is advantageous, providing control and helping the patient to monitor his or her own speech. Direct voice therapy should not continue for an indefinite period, but only as long as needed to achieve the two goals of treatment: counseling about realistic goals and eliminating and/or lessening the undesirable symptoms.

### Counseling

The voice therapist discusses the where, why, and how of vocal abuse or misuse with the patient. The goal is to help the patient eliminate or reduce bad habits such as throat clearing, coughing, and excessive speaking. Vocal abuse also includes smoking, drinking alcohol, and, consuming caffeine. Certain medications, such as decongestants and diuretics, may cause or aggravate dryness, which in turn can cause vocal problems. More subtle vocal misuse is associated with excessive telephone use or with carrying on conversations in noisy surroundings such as clamorous restaurants.

## Direct Strategies for Working on the Voice

1 Use an amplifier (microphone) and a tape recorder.

2 Develop more effective breathing patterns for speaking by working on pausing and phrasing.

3 Use relaxation techniques to reduce head, neck, and bodily tension.

4 Eliminate the hard glottal attack when initiating speech. This is a way of speaking in which one "punches out" words that begin with high pressure consonants such as p, t, k, ch. This results in the vocal cords slamming together and irritation.

### Helpful Suggestions

1 Sipping water provides temporary relief for voice problems caused by dryness.

2 Using a humidifier at home helps keep air moist.

3 Nasal breathing is preferable to open-mouth breathing. While engaging in relaxation exercises, breathe in and out through the nose.

4 Since the salivary glands in Sjogren's syndrome patients produce only a limited amount of saliva, the stimulation provided by chewing sugarless gum may improve production.

5 Avoid clearing the throat by sipping water, sucking on a hard sugarless candy, or simply swallowing. If clearing the throat cannot be prevented, using an "h" sound or humming will soften the attack on the vocal cords.

6 When patients have difficulty getting a word out, they may fear that they are losing their voices totally. Although complete loss of voice is rare, the emotional element of fear affects voice production. When having trouble getting a word out, try an easy-onset "h" word such as Hi, a humming sound, or a laugh, using this technique the vocal cords come together without tension.

7 Use a nasal douche before going to bed. Keep a humidifier on while sleeping. Open-mouth breathing during sleep dries out the throat and larynx.

8  When speaking to a group, as opposed to conversing socially with one or two friends, speak for a limited time and use a microphone. Speak in a small room, if possible, so that the audience will be close by.

9  Keep a vocal log, charting daily voice use in various situations.

# 23 What You Should Know About Medication Use

WITH THE ADVANCES in drug development, many diseases can now be managed or cured. Advances such as the discovery of penicillin, polio vaccine, and, most recently, the chickenpox vaccine improve the quality of life of most people today. Like a double-edged sword, however, drugs have harmful as well as beneficial effects if not used judiciously. It is not always possible to prevent all the side effects that can occur with drug use; however, certain general guidelines should be followed to ensure safe use. These general guidelines and important information regarding side effects and drug interactions are presented below, followed by specific information for patients with Sjogren's syndrome.

## Checklist for Appropriate Drug Use

1   Keep a list of drugs that you are currently taking and have taken in the past (prescription and over-the-counter products), including the name and strength of each drug.

2   Keep a list of how often and how much of each drug you take.

3   Keep a note of when you started or stopped taking a drug.

4   Any time you get a new drug, ask your doctor and/or pharmacist what the drug is used for, what it does, what common and/or dangerous side effects can occur, and when you should seek medical advice if a side effect does occur.

5  Bring your medication list to the doctor's office. This is especially important if you see several different doctors.

6  Try to have all your prescriptions filled at one pharmacy. This will ensure that the pharmacist has a profile of all of your medications and will help to avoid potentially harmful drug interactions.

7  Always follow the doctor's and/or pharmacist's instructions on how to take your medication.

8  Take all of the medication prescribed even if you are feeling better.

9  If you have any questions about your medications, always ask the physician or pharmacist. There are no dumb questions.

10 Flush outdated or discontinued medications down the toilet.

## The "Don't" List of Drug Use

1  Never use someone else's medication even if you have the same symptoms.

2  Never give your medication to someone else.

3  Children are not little adults; do not give them a "small amount" of an adult medication unless instructed to do so by your doctor.

4  Do not abruptly stop taking a chronic medication until you discuss it with your doctor.

5  Do not take a double dose of a medication because you missed a dose unless instructed to do so by your doctor or pharmacist.

6  Never store medications in your bathroom cabinet or any cabinet in which there are dramatic changes in temperature or humidity. Such changes causes medications to break down faster.

7  Never keep medications where children can easily get to them. Don't forget about young visitors such as grandchildren.

8  If you are taking medications for a chronic illness, do not take any other medications or herbal remedies without discussing them with your doctor or pharmacist.

## Side Effects

Side effects can occur despite the most careful use of drugs. Many side effects are unavoidable and must be tolerated when the beneficial effects of the drug are needed. For example, persons with hay fever would not want to give up the beneficial effects of antihistamines. Yet, for some of these drugs, drowsiness is an unavoidable side effect. Many side effects do not pose a great risk to patients by themselves. However, if a person is taking an antihistamine that causes drowsiness, although the drowsiness itself is not dangerous, it would be dangerous for the patient to drive. Therefore, warning labels on over-the-counter and prescription drugs are needed (e.g., do not take with alcohol, do not drive).

Some side effects, such as a change in the color of urine, are harmless, while others, such as dizziness, are dangerous. Ask your physician or pharmacist what common side effects occur with the medication, which ones are dangerous, what symptoms to watch out for, and when you should seek medical attention if side effects do occur. In some cases, a change in the dose is all that is needed to solve the problem.

## Allergic Reactions

Allergic reactions can range in severity from a simple rash to an anaphylactic (hypotensive) reaction from which the patient can die. Regardless of its severity, it is important for your doctor and pharmacist to know if you have had an allergic reaction. One of the main reasons is to avoid using the drug that caused the problem, but even more important, to avoid using similar drugs. For example, if a patient had an anaphylactic reaction to "Penicillin VK," other penicillin drugs, such as amoxicillin, ampicillin, and ticarcillin, should be avoided. In addition, a similar group of antibiotics known as cephalosporins should probably not be prescribed for this patient. The severity of the reaction determines whether similar drugs can or cannot be used. Therefore, if you had an allergic reaction or any side effect, you should keep a record of the following information:

1  The drug that caused the problem (both the brand and generic names) and how much you took.

2  The symptoms you had (e.g., problems breathing, rash).

3 After you started taking the drug, how long it took before the reaction occurred.

4 Whether you had to stop taking the drug whether or the dose was changed.

5 If the doctor instructed you to stop taking the drug, how long it took before the symptoms disappeared.

6 How long it has been since you last took this medication.

In addition, you should ask the doctor or pharmacist what other drugs to avoid taking. These include prescription and over-the-counter drugs that you take by mouth, lotions, ointments, creams, sprays, inhalers, and those that are given by injection.

## What You Should Know About Drug Interactions

Drug interactions refer to the effects that occur when (1) two or more drugs are taken by the same patient; (2) two or more drugs are taken at the same time; (3) a drug and food are taken together; or (4) a drug interferes with a laboratory test. If two or more drugs with the same side effects are taken, the side effects can be intensified. For example, a patient who is taking an antihistamine and a sedative may experience more drowsiness than either of those drugs would cause alone.

Almost all drugs are eliminated from the body through the kidneys or liver. Some drugs have the ability to change the rate at which other drugs are eliminated. For example, one drug used for the treatment of gout is given to patients who are being treated with penicillin for gonorrhea because it decreases the rate of elimination of penicillin. This allows penicillin to stay in the body for a longer period of time to fight the infection. This is an example of a drug interaction that is used for the benefit of the patient. In other cases, an adjustment of the drug dose is all that is needed to manage drug interaction, and both drugs can be used by the patient.

When two drugs are taken at the same time, one drug may have the ability to either increase or decrease the absorption of the second drug into the bloodstream, or to increase or decrease the time it takes the second drug to be absorbed. Calcium can bind tetracycline (an antibiotic) in the stomach, allowing a smaller amount of tetracycline to be absorbed. In essence, the patient is getting a smaller dose, and the drug may thus not be as effective. In such cases, two drugs should not be taken at the same time. Whether a drug that changes the rate of absorption is important depends on the purpose of the drugs involved. For example, if you take a pain killer for a headache, you probably would not want another drug to slow down the time it takes to get an adequate amount of the pain killer into your bloodstream.

When food is taken with a drug, it may decrease either the amount of drug that is absorbed or the rate of absorption. As in the case of two drugs taken at the same time, the rate of absorption may or may not be important, depending on the drugs involved. Changes in the amount of drug that is absorbed may also be important, depending on how big the change is. Dairy products should not be used while taking tetracycline because they contain calcium, which reduces absorption of the drug. For some drugs, ingestion of certain foods can lead to harmful side effects. The most common example of this type of interaction involves monoamine oxidase (MAO) inhibitors (used in the treatment of depression). These patients must avoid foods such as aged cheese, red wine, and smoked or pickled meats because they contain substances known as tyramines; MAO inhibitors stop the breakdown of these substances in the body. Patients who eat such foods while taking MAO inhibitors can develop a sudden increase in blood pressure that is potentially very dangerous.

Lastly, drugs can affect the results of certain laboratory tests. Some drugs can cause a laboratory test to become positive when it really should not be, indicating that a medical problem may be present. Others can cause a test to be negative when it really should be positive, indicating that there is no problem. How critical this problem is depends on the test. Your doctor and laboratory technicians should know what drugs may interfere with laboratory tests and how that situation should be managed.

In summary, drug interactions may be used for the patient's benefit, may cause the patient harm, or may have no real effect at all. Even though a drug interaction may exist, it does not mean that the two drugs cannot be used together. It may simply mean adjusting the doses or just not taking both drugs at the same time. The effects of drug interactions are most commonly seen when a new drug is added or stopped while you are taking other drugs. This is the time when you should carefully watch to see if a drug interaction develops. As with side effects, you should ask your doctor or pharmacist if a drug interaction is expected to occur. If so, find out what symptoms you should watch out for or how you should manage that interaction. Lastly, it is important to provide your doctor and pharmacist with a list of prescription and over-the-counter medications that you are taking so that they can determine if a drug interaction may occur.

## Patients with Sjogren's Syndrome

The majority of persons with Sjogren's syndrome have symptoms related to a decrease in tear and saliva production. Therefore, it is important for such patients to avoid using drugs that are likely to cause dryness of the mouth and eyes.

Drugs with anticholinergic effects decrease saliva and tear production. Examples of such drugs are antihistamines, certain antipsychotic drugs, tranquilizers, some blood pressure medications, and antidepressants. It may not be possible to avoid their use; however, a doctor may be able to choose a drug within a particular group of drugs with the least potential to cause dryness. If this option does not exist, you may need to use additional doses of artificial tears or saliva and drink more fluids. It is best to inform the doctor and pharmacist that you have Sjogren's syndrome if they are not aware of it already. Ask about the potential for these drugs to decrease fluid production and how the problem should be managed.

In summary, if these general guidelines are followed, if patients take responsibility for the medications they are using, and if health professionals fulfill their professional obligation of adequately informing and counseling patients, drugs can be used safely. The most important things that patients can do are to have information about their drugs, keep good records, and provide this information to the health professionals who are taking care of them.

John V. Donlon, Jr., MD

# 24 Anesthetic Management of Patients with Sjogren's Syndrome

KNOWLEDGE OF Sjogren's syndrome can help anesthesiologists plan a proper general anesthetic, avoiding discomfort and complications for the patient. The most common postoperative problems associated with Sjogren's syndrome are burning eyes (corneal dryness, abrasion) and sore throats.

Anesthetic care plans for Sjogren's syndrome patients should include the following:

1 A prolonged NPO (nothing by mouth) status is not necessary. Patients may have clear liquids until 2 hours before surgery.

2 Omit drying agents such as atropine, diphenhydramine, glycopyrrolate, and phenergan.

3 Add a humidifier to the rebreathing system. The $CO_2$ absorber absorbs moisture, and anesthetic gases are dry.

4 Lubricate the eyes every 30 minutes to prevent corneal dryness and abrasions. Tape the eyelids gently closed and avoid pressure on them. General anesthesia itself causes decreased tear production over and above the effect of Sjogren's syndrome.

5 Lubricate endotracheal tubes (ETTs) or laryngeal mask airways (LMAs) well. LMAs avoid tracheal irritation. Dry airways are more likely to have thick mucous plugs.

6 Beware of carious teeth and thin oral mucosa. Use a dental guard.

7 Perform the laryngoscopy and place the ETT or LMA very carefully.

8 The rheumatoid arthritis associated with Sjogren's syndrome can affect the cervical spine, making it fragile. The temporal mandibular joints and arytenoids may be involved in the rheumatic process, making intubation difficult. Consideration should be given to fiberoptic intubation, use of a smaller endotracheal tube or LMA as indicated by each situation.

9 Steroid treatment schedules should be continued and supplemented with intravenous doses during surgery if necessary.

10 The operating room should be kept warmer than usual due to some Sjogren's patients' susceptibility to attacks of Raynaud's phenomenon precipitated by cold.

11 Consider that patients with Sjogren's syndrome may have mild renal dysfunction and adjust drug dosages accordingly.

12 In the recovery room, provide humidified oxygen and avoid pain medications such as meperidine, which have a vagolytic effect and may contribute to mucosal dryness. The patient should be permitted to suck on ice chips as soon as it is practical, and the patient's room should have a bedside humidifier.

Depending on the nature of the surgical procedure, a local or regional anesthetic technique may be possible. This should be discussed with the surgeon and anesthesiologist.

During the preoperative interview, the patient should be reassured that the anesthesiologist is aware of the implications of Sjogren's syndrome and will follow the guidelines outlined above to achieve a pleasant, safe anesthesia with a minimum of discomfort or complications.

# 25 Living with Sjogren's Syndrome

WHEN FACED WITH the knowledge that life will change due to Sjogren's syndrome, each person responds differently to the issues of change, loss, and uncertainty. Whether you have just been diagnosed with Sjogren's syndrome or have had it for some time, there are always ways that you can improve your life. For any person with Sjogren's syndrome, emotional needs may be just as important as the physical management of the disorder. The goal is not simply to live with Sjogren's syndrome, but to live well with it.

Living successfully with any problem, such as a chronic disease, involves three important steps: understanding as much as possible about the problem, implementing any changes that can make your life more comfortable and efficient, and learning to cope with and adapt to anything that you cannot change.

With regard to these three steps, hopefully, this book gives you a greater understanding of Sjogren's syndrome, as well as current treatments, suggestions, and tips to improve your physical health. There are always ways to improve your ability to change, handle, or compensate for the symptoms of Sjogren's syndrome. What about the things that you cannot change? This is where the art of successful coping comes in. Undeniably, this requires considerable strength and hard work. Remember that you are neither helpless nor alone in this effort, and that trained professionals, counseling centers, and support groups are available. Wonderful coping strategies have been developed to help you deal with things you cannot change. The following sections discuss some of the strategies that have been used by professionals to help those with Sjogren's syndrome adjust and cope.

## Identify Your Concerns

As an exercise, simply asking yourself important direct questions can be a powerful start. Often the act of writing these questions down and answering them opens the door to the lifelong process of successful coping. In what ways does Sjogren's syndrome affect you? Have your relationships changed? How? What do you do differently that is related to Sjogren's syndrome? What thoughts continue to trouble you? What situations can you not change? These questions arise from your personal experience. The answers to the questions will help you identify your concerns clearly and start the process of improvement and skillful coping.

Once you have identified your concerns and areas for improvement, you can start to select helpful strategies. This chapter will discuss strategies that fall into four important categories: using relaxation techniques, improving your thinking, enhancing your support system, and considering professional help and support groups.

## Use Relaxation Procedures Regularly

Relaxation techniques can be an important part of your efforts to live better with Sjogren's syndrome. They are important for two reasons:

1 To reduce the physiological and psychological impact of the symptoms (either physical or emotional)

2 To eliminate or control situations, circumstances, or stressors that may make it more difficult for you to handle the symptoms

Relaxation techniques can be used in two important ways: preventively and curatively. Preventive use of the relaxation techniques gets your body accustomed to the process and builds up your confidence. This reduces the likelihood of experiencing extreme stress responses. Curative use of the techniques allows you to maintain or regain control at the first sign of a problem.

Why do relaxation techniques work? Relaxation is incompatible with tension. Learning how to respond automatically to an anxiety-provoking situation with a relaxation technique reduces the intensity of anxiety immediately.

In order to make relaxation an automatic, positive response, practice relaxation techniques frequently. The more you practice, the more your body becomes conditioned to these comfortable, healthy feelings and the more quickly you benefit from them.

There are many different types of relaxation techniques. Here's an effective technique called the Quick Release that is easy to learn. Read the directions completely before beginning this procedure.

Close your eyes, take a breath, and hold it while tensing as many muscles as you can concentrate on (without straining). Hold this breath and keep your body tense for approximately 6 seconds. Then let your breath out in a "whoosh" and allow the tension to flow out of your body. Let your body go limp. Keeping your eyes closed, breathe rhythmically and comfortably for approximately 20 seconds. Repeat this 6-second–20-second cycle twice.

This entire procedure takes less than 2 minutes. Initially, you should attempt to practice it at least five times throughout the day. In addition, any time you feel anxiety and would like to gain the feeling of control, the "Quick Release" can help. Of course, three repetitions are not necessarily best. You be the judge.

### Work On Your Thinking

Many people with Sjogren's syndrome handle their disorder well because they are able to think appropriately, constructively, and realistically about their condition. Others may have a much harder time because of their inability to control their thinking.

The difference between being happy and unhappy is not whether you experience negative thoughts. Rather, the difference is determined by how successful you are in dealing with the negative thoughts that do occur. This is an area in which the help of a skilled professional may be invaluable. However, here are a few suggestions for working on your thoughts by yourself.

### Reword Your Negative Thoughts

If Sjogren's syndrome leads to negative emotions such as fear, anger, or depression, you should begin to address your internal dialogue (i.e., your own thoughts). It is important to develop constructive techniques to change the way you think. For example, you could learn how to restructure (i.e., reword) negative thoughts by turning them into realistic positives, a process called cognitive restructuring. First, start to identify and reword your negative thinking. (For example, you might think, "I'm never going to feel any better.") Replace inappropriate and counterproductive words with more positive and realistic ones. (Using this example, you might ask yourself, "How do I know I'm not going to feel any better? Isn't it possible that I could feel better? And as long as it *is* possible to feel better, why should I convince myself that I won't?") Cognitive restructuring helps you do two things: recognize the negative or inappropriate thoughts and improve your approach to and attitude toward problems and emotions.

### Think Clearly and Positively

The quality of your thoughts can help you feel better even if you cannot change anything going on around you. Try to stay in the here and now by using the present tense to frame your thoughts. Your spoken words and inner expressions should positively address your situation. Try to avoid negative terms such as useless, tragic, can't, and impossible.

If you feel your thoughts are not clear and concise, *stop!* Begin again with simple statements that are positive. Once you develop clear, positive thoughts, write them down. Read them, and continue using and repeating this process.

### Use Positive Statements to Describe Yourself

Try to characterize yourself in positively worded statements that may be stated out loud or in thought. For example, you might say, "I have Sjogren's syndrome, but I'm still a capable and responsible individual." Repeat these positive statements to yourself frequently. The more you do this, the more you will start to believe them. As long as these statements are realistic, this technique will be effective.

### Avoid Comparisons with Others

People unnecessarily compare themselves to others with regard to any characteristic. Unhappily, it is not unusual for those with Sjogren's syndrome to compare themselves to persons who do not have the condition. You may be more fragile emotionally than you realize. Criticizing yourself can often make you feel that you will fall short in comparison to others. Realistically, there will always be people who are better, as well as worse, no matter what characteristics are under the critical eye. Remind yourself of this when you find yourself making comparisons. Use this as a reason to stop this harmful process.

### Improve Your Support System

Nobody likes problems, but it can be much easier to deal with them if you have supportive family members or friends behind you. All too often, relationships break down because of a lack of understanding or communication. Let's discuss two ways of improving your relationships: education and communication.

### Educate Family and Friends

All too often, problems arise with those who are important to you because they don't understand how Sjogren's syndrome affects you. Their lack of knowledge or understanding can cause a strain in the relationship. Sit down and talk with them, keeping two main goals in mind:

1 First, try to educate them about Sjogren's syndrome (this book can certainly help!) to make them more sensitive to how it affects you. (Anticipate, though, that if they have already had difficulty understanding Sjogren's syndrome, not much may change.)

2 If you can't change their level of understanding, attitude, or support, at least ask them to allow you to deal with Sjogren's syndrome in ways that are best for you. For example, if you must frequently stop what you're doing to lubricate your eyes, ask them not to be critical or rush you; let them either help you or avoid saying anything that might be counterproductive.

### Improve Communication

Good communication is the key to good interpersonal relationships. Often, problems in relationships occur when communication breaks down. An essential way to improve strained relationships is to improve communication. If you're having difficulty living with Sjogren's syndrome, you can help by taking the time to discuss your problems with important people in your life. Here are a few suggestions for improving communication.

### Phrase Your Comments Constructively

It may not be helpful to say angrily, "I can't stand the fact that you have no idea what I'm going through." Many communication problems occur because your message is not being delivered in a helpful way. Think before you speak. Say things the way you'd want to hear them from others. For example, it would be better to say, "It's probably impossible for you to totally understand how Sjogren's syndrome can be a problem. Let me try to explain it to you." This can make others more receptive to what you have to say.

### Be a Better Listener

Better listeners become better communicators. Ask your friends and family how they feel about an issue. Don't interrupt when they are expressing their feelings or opinions. Be sure you're fully aware of what they're saying. You may even want to restate their comments in your own words to show that you understand what they have just said. This will also show them how you'd like them to listen to you in the future.

### Change Your Perspective

If you are totally wrapped up in your own point of view, you will have a difficult time understanding someone else's feelings or comments. Try to see the problem through the other person's eyes. This will help you explain your point of view far more effectively.

### Strive to Improve Support from Family and Friends

What reactions would you like from people around you when something is bothering you? How would you like them to express their support? Have you told them, in a way that they can understand, what you need to hear and feel from them? When you can answer these questions, you will get some ideas about what and how to communicate with those who are important to you.

## Consider Psychological Counseling

Although self-help procedures are useful for some individuals, with Sjogren's syndrome, many others are best served by working with a qualified professional specializing in counseling those with medical problems. If you decide that this method may be helpful, speak to your doctor or another reputable person to obtain the name of an expert in this area.

There are many ways professional treatment can be helpful. Below, we discuss three of them: learning how to deal better with your feelings, using strategies discussed in this chapter more effectively, and helping your family better understand what you're going through.

### Get Help with Your Feelings

Talking to somebody who is objective and supportive can be very reassuring. Professionals can help you put your feelings in perspective, discussing different ways of looking at an issue that you may have considered in only one emotionally unpleasant way. Professionals can help you learn effective coping strategies to deal with any problems, physical or emotional. They can suggest different actions you can take or different ways of thinking about things you can't change.

### Get Help Through Effective Techniques

The therapeutic techniques the professional uses depend on what emotional reactions or problems need improvement. There are a variety of techniques, each suited to different situations and problems. As described above, cognitive techniques can teach you how to reduce your negativity and use more realistically positive thoughts.

### Get Help with Family Relationships

Of course, counseling may be helpful in working with family members. Professionals can help both you and any family members who are affected by your condition. Therapists themselves need to have a good grasp of the potential difficulties due to Sjogren's syndrome in order to help you live with it successfully.

### Attend Support Groups

People with Sjogren's syndrome need to know that they are not alone. Joining a structured self-help or support group may be very helpful in living successfully with Sjogren's syndrome. Participants often share how they handle various problems. These groups provide a forum for the exchange of feelings and ideas, as well as suggestions on how to cope better.

Sjogren's syndrome support organizations also bring patients and families together and provide a lot of beneficial information. They can help educate family members, giving them a chance to get some support of their own.

## A Coping Conclusion

There are many ways in which Sjogren's syndrome can affect you. Your goal, regardless, is to learn to lead a happy, healthy, and productive life. Accordingly, learning how to cope with Sjogren's syndrome as successfully as possible is the key to a good quality of life.

Elaine K. Harris, MA

Updated by Rita M. May M.Ed
and Alexis Stegemann, BA

# 26 Tips for Daily Living with Sjogren's Syndrome and Some Frequently Asked Questions

AT THE SJOGREN'S SYNDROME FOUNDATION, a day does not go by when someone does not call asking for a recommendation of a product that will alleviate a profoundly bothersome symptom. We do our best to listen and learn. Our dedicated members keep us informed regarding their personal experiences with Sjogren's syndrome, convincing us that the management of the numerous life-altering aspects of pervasive sicca (dryness) symptoms is the challenge of living with Sjogren's syndrome. The magnitude of the dryness caused by Sjogren's syndrome demands that a patient create a personal daily regimen to control the symptoms and remain comfortable.

The number of preparations available for relief of the symptoms of dryness grows each day. One has only to read the advertisements in health magazines or the Sunday supplement of any newspaper to see the vast array of products available. Judging the effectiveness of over-the-counter products is the job of each patient. With an eye to safety and a healthy dose of common sense, however, we at the Sjogren's Syndrome Foundation would like to pass on a few of the tips that have proved to help our members. Many of the following suggestions have appeared in issues of *The Moisture Seekers Newsletter*.

## Some Tips for Daily Living
### Tips for Oral Comfort
(See Chapters 6 and 21)

*Beginning at Your Lips*

- Keep a thin coat of oil- or petroleum-based lubricant on your lips; even shortening used in cooking provides appropriate moisturizing. (*Note*: lipstick is a petroleum-based lubricant and provides this needed protection well.)

- Break a vitamin E capsule inside your mouth, especially before retiring for the night. This provides a protective, soothing coating that is unlikely to evaporate.

*On to Your Mouth and Tender Mucous Membranes*

- Artificial salivas or saliva substitutes may provide temporary relief from the sensation of dryness in the mouth.

- Frequent, small sips of water hydrate the mouth and gastrointestinal tract. Sucking on ice chips has a similar effect.

- Drink sugar-free beverages.

- Keep a carafe of water at your bedside for dryness during the night or on awakening.

- Chewing helps stimulate the production of saliva in salivary glands that have residual function. Chew sugarless gum.

- Chewing gum containing Xylitol (a sugar substitute) can produce a cariostatic (cavity-inhibiting) effect.

- Suck on large fruit pits (e.g., prune, peach) or sugarless hard candies.

- Never sleep with gum or with anything else in the mouth. Aspiration of any substance during sleep can be dangerous.

- Avoid spicy and acidic foods, as they irritate oral tissue.

- Use self-adhesive postage stamps. When sealing envelopes or other non-self-adhesive containers, use a damp sponge.

- Avoid coffee, tea, alcohol, and caffeinated beverages. These are dehydrating, and many patients report increased dryness after drinking them.

- Use a mild saline mouthwash to break up thick, mucous-like saliva in the mouth.

- Combat oral candidiasis (yeast infections) by sucking on tablets that combat vaginal yeast infections. These do not contain sugar and usually dissolve in the mouth in 15 to 30 minutes (not very tasty, but they are effective).

- Avoid regular oral troches and oral suspensions, as they contain sugar.

### Saving Your Tooth Enamel

- Maintain meticulous dental hygiene.

- Brush the teeth immediately before and after eating. Brushing before eating helps to eliminate bacteria in the mouth that attach to food particles, causing dental decay.

- Floss daily.

- Avoid sticky, sugary foods.

- Drink milk when tolerated. Milk does not remineralize teeth, but it contains a substance that coats the teeth to prevent caries.

- If you chew vitamin C tablets, brush your teeth immediately afterward or at least rinse your mouth thoroughly. Vitamin C contains sufficient acid to start to dissolve tooth enamel in a compromised mouth.

- See your dentist at least three times per year to check on and, if necessary, treat caries in the enamel and at the roots of your teeth.

- Use toothpaste containing fluoride.

- Use a pH-balanced mouthwash to sweeten and lower acidity in the mouth: dissolve one-fourth of a teaspoon of baking soda in one-fourth of a cup of warm water. This is helpful if foods or beverages leave an unpleasant aftertaste.

- Ask your dentist to apply a fluoride varnish to your teeth.

- Special toothpastes and gels are available for anyone with dry mouth. These can be helpful to Sjogren's syndrome patients when used in a conscientious program of dental hygiene.

### *Relieving Pain in the Parotid Salivary Gland Area*

- Gently massage the area just below the bottom of the earlobe with the fleshy part of your index and middle fingers. Go forward toward the end of the jawbone, slightly downward and over the jawbone, and then up again toward the tip of the earlobe. This sometimes helps to dislodge a mucous plug in a duct, relieving the pain caused by a blockage.

## Tips to Manage Nasal and Airway Dryness
(See Chapters 7 and 9)

A moisturizing regimen for the respiratory tract sounds unusual, but that is just what is needed to avoid some of the painful effects of a dry environment. Nasal cracking and bleeding, as well as coughing due to irritated bronchi and trachea, can be avoided to some extent by adding water vapor to the air you breathe; every droplet helps.

- Use a humidifier. It can be installed in a furnace or purchased as a stand-alone model.

- Both air conditioning and heating lower ambient humidity, so use your humidifier year round.

- Clean humidifiers and air conditioners regularly and properly to prevent mildew and mold from forming inside the mechanisms.

- Keep nasal passages moist and lubricated by using a saline nasal spray or gel at the base of the nostril.

- Sleeping can be problematic for sensitive airways. A crockpot filled with water and kept "on" all day is a safe way to moisturize the air, especially in the bedroom.

- Keep your bedroom as cool as possible.

- A baby vaporizer, with either cold or warm steam, can be an effective room humidifier.

- Avoid the use of petroleum-based products other than at the tip of the nostril; use inside the nasal passages can result in aspiration into the lung.

- Vitamin E, suspended in fine oil in caplet form, makes an excellent external lubricant. Use only at the rim of the nostril.

- For severe sinus and nasal dryness, try a nasal douche. This also helps soften and moisten accumulated dry mucus. Irrigate your nose daily with a mild saline solution (one-fourth of a teaspoon of salt to one cup of water) using a commercial nasal douche device. A nasal irrigator (sold in the baby products section of pharmacies) is a good alternative to a nasal douche.

- Steam inhalers can be used effectively to clear your nose and throat. The steam can soften accumulated dry nasal mucus deep inside for easier expulsion. Facial saunas can also be used for this purpose.

- Care should be taken when removing dried or crusted mucus from the nose. Use a moistened cotton swab just inside the nostrils to help remove this mucus.

- Try using a soft cervical collar (the type worn for neck injuries) while you sleep. The collar keeps your mouth from dropping open during sleep, thus preventing dryness from mouth breathing.

### When a Nosebleed Occurs

- Let gravity help. Sit up to lower the pressure in the veins of your nose.

- Keep your head tilted forward a bit to stop blood from running into your throat.

- Pinch the fleshy part of your nose between the bridge and nostrils with the thumb and index fingers for 5 to 10 minutes. *Note:* application of ice is not believed to stop the bleeding; rather, it is the direct pressure that does the trick.

- If pressure alone does not stop the bleeding, wet a cotton or tissue plug with a decongestant nasal solution, insert this gently into the nostril, and reapply pressure.

- After the bleeding stops, take special care not to blow your nose except very gently. If necessary, sneeze with your mouth open. Finally, avoid strenuous sports for a few days.

- Remember to lubricate your nose and take special care when flying in airplanes.

- If nosebleeds are persistent or/and frequent, see your doctor to determine the cause and the appropriate treatment.

## Tips for Living with Dry Eyes
(See Chapter 5)

- Although not essential for sterility, it is advisable to keep nonpreserved artificial tears cool.

- Lunch boxes containing coolant that hardens in the freezer can be used to keep tears cool when traveling.

- Apply warm compresses to your eyes each morning for a few minutes to soothe dry, irritated tissues at the edge of the eyelid.

- If neck stiffness occurs on arising in the morning, keep artificial tears at your bedside. While still lying down, you can instill drops into your eye.

- Frequent users (more than four times per day) of artificial tears should avoid many preservative-containing products, since their prolonged use causes a buildup in the ocular tissue or provokes allergy-like reactions. However, preservatives that oxidize (hydrogen peroxide) on the ocular surface do not build up.

- Keep your eyelids clean with lid wipes to help prevent eye infections.

- Moisture chamber glasses can be made for you by trained optometrists or opticians and may even be worn by persons who do not wear prescription eyeglasses. Moisture chambers decrease tear film evaporation by reducing air circulation immediately around the eyes.

- Wearing swim or ski goggles at night may help retain moisture around the eye.

- Wraparound sunglasses/goggles with side shields that can be worn over prescription glasses are available through ophthalmologists, optometrists, and opticians.

- To clean the eyelids and lashes, wipe them with special eyelid scrub washes for dry eyes. A less expensive method is to wipe the lids with a mixture of equal parts of warm water and baby shampoo; this may cause irritation to susceptible individuals.

### Treating Blepharitis

- Use a first-aid gel pack that has been heated and wrapped in thick washcloths as a warm compress. Lie down, apply the pack to your eyes, and relax.

## Tips for More Comfortable Skin

- Avoid antibacterial or abrasive soaps.

- Use soaps with added emollients or oils.

- Bathe no more than once a day. If you take tub baths, soak in the tub for 10 to 15 minutes to hydrate your skin.

- When you take a shower or a bath, do not dry off completely. Leave a film of moisture and then generously apply lubricant. Generally, creams are more effective and longer-lasting moisturizers than lotions.

- When using bath oils, apply them directly to the skin. This avoids an oily ring in the tub that could cause falls.

- For dry skin with thick scaling, use emollients containing urea, lactate, or salicylic acid, which cause the skin to peel by breaking up the dead skin and helping it to slough off. They also smooth and soften thick, rough, or scaly skin.

- Diet has no effect on the amount of moisture your skin receives. Except in extreme circumstances, such as malnutrition or severe dehydration, what you eat is not related to your skin's condition in any way.

- Hard water may aggravate skin dryness; if you live in a hard water area, try installing a water conditioner to your water supply system.

- Avoid using fabric softener sheets. These may cause contact dermatitis in sensitive persons. Liquid fabric softener may not have this effect.

- On all skin exposed to sunlight, use at least a #15 (sun protection factor) sunscreen as a moisturizer.

- Before swimming, apply a moistener to your skin.

## Some Advice When Taking Medication or Pills
If you have difficulty swallowing pills:

- Cut pills in half (many of them are scored) and take each piece separately with plenty of water. A commercial pill cutter will help avoid sharp edges that can damage delicate tissue. Do not break up capsules.

- Let gravity help. Sit or stand up when taking pills. Stay in an upright position for at least 2 or 3 minutes.

- Swallow some water to lubricate your mouth and throat before putting a pill or capsule in your mouth.

- Place the pill or capsule as far back as possible in the middle of your tongue without gagging.

- Wash medicine down with at least 4 ounces of water. If possible, drink another half glass of water 5 minutes later.

- If a pill gets stuck in your throat, eat several bites of a soft food such as banana or bread and then drink some water. The bulk will help push the pill down.

- Immediately after taking a liquid medication, rinse your mouth with water to reduce the acidity from the medication, thus preventing possible mouth ulcers from forming.

## Tips for Travel
### Airplane Travel

The relative humidity in an airplane is very low; therefore, it is important to fortify yourself with liquids and moisturizers.

### Nose
- Apply emollients to the edges of your nostrils. If you have a stuffy nose, use medication before entering the plane.

- Spray saline into your nose frequently during the trip.

### Eyes
- Swim or ski goggles help preserve moisture, especially while sleeping. Moisture chamber glasses, if worn, should not be removed during the flight.

- Use artificial tears more frequently than usual.

- If you are carrying a large quantity of your favorite artificial tears on a trip abroad, request a note from your physician explaining your need for this product to facilitate your passage through customs.

- If your eyes hurt, request a hot washcloth to put over your eyes. This is particularly important if you suffer from blepharitis. (It is a good idea to keep a clean washcloth handy for use throughout your trip.)

- If warm-water compresses do not help, try using ice chips wrapped in a washcloth.

**Mouth**

- Use sugarless gum or suck on sugarless candy to keep your mouth moist.

- Ask the flight attendant for a few ice cubes; suck on them to stimulate salivary secretions and provide moisture throughout the flight.

*Car, Train, or Bus Travel*

For prolonged travel, most of the information on plane travel can be adapted to travel on the road, particularly if you're a passenger. Remember, if you are driving, do not use eye ointment because it causes blurring. Also, as a driver, you should take frequent breaks to instill eye drops before your eyes begin to hurt.

Smoke-free environments are becoming the norm in the United States. Such guestrooms are now available on request at most motels and hotels. Fortunately, all U.S. airline flights are now smoke-free. This is particularly beneficial to Sjogren's syndrome patients, who do not need any additional irritation to the eyes or respiratory tract.

## Frequently Asked Questions

Throughout each day, the Foundation answers many questions regarding Sjogren's syndrome. Reprinted here are the answers to those that are frequently asked. Insightful and accurate answers to all the questions listed below are available in this book.

### Is Sjogren's Syndrome Contagious?

Sjogren's syndrome is not a contagious disease. It cannot be passed from one person to another in any way. Sjogren's syndrome is an autoimmune disease, as is rheumatoid arthritis; that is, the body's immune system attacks itself, damaging the moisture-producing glands of the body.

### What Kind of Doctor Should I See If I Think I Might Have Sjogren's Syndrome?

The physician most likely to diagnose Sjogren's syndrome is a rheumatologist. However, any trained, knowledgeable healthcare professional may diagnose and treat Sjogren's syndrome.

## Is Sjogren's Syndrome a Hereditary Disease?

At this time, there is no evidence that Sjogren's syndrome is hereditary. However, some persons seem to have a predisposition to autoimmune diseases.

## Can Sjogren's Syndrome Be Cured?

As yet, there is no cure for Sjogren's syndrome. The Sjogren's Syndrome Foundation, through its fellowship grants and summer student research grants, encourages research to find a cure and provide effective treatments.

## If Sjogren's Syndrome Is an Autoimmune Disease, Is It the Same as Acquired Immunodeficiency Syndrome (AIDS) or Human Immunodeficiency Virus (HIV)?

No, this is not the same type of disease. In AIDS, the immune system is compromised by a viral infection and becomes underactive or inactive, no longer able to protect the body from opportunistic (infectious) diseases. In Sjogren's syndrome, the immune system is overactive because the body's immune cells react to its own tissue as foreign.

## Who Gets Sjogren's Syndrome?

Currently, 90 percent of the known patients are women. Men are less likely than women to be diagnosed with Sjogren's syndrome. Children are rarely diagnosed with the condition. Sjogren's syndrome appears to strike all races and ethnic groups equally.

## What Can I Expect If I Have Been Diagnosed with Sjogren's Syndrome?

Each person with Sjogren's syndrome has a unique medical history. Some patients experience periods of good health with occasional flare-ups; some find that their symptoms plateau; in others, their symptoms go into remission; in still others, their symptoms become progressively worse. There is no defined course of the disease.

## What Can Be Done to Help?

For many persons with a chronic disease, learning about their illness empowers them to take control of their lives. The Sjogren's Syndrome Foundation provides educational materials to patients and their families about Sjogren's syndrome and about how to cope with a chronic illness.

### Why Did It Take Years for Me to Get a Diagnosis of Sjogren's Syndrome?

This is unfortunately the case for many patients. A recent study found that diagnosis took on average 6.3 years from a Sjogren's patients first reported symptoms. Doctors' unawareness is not the sole reason for the delay. The blood tests for autoantibodies are not specific enough to identify the different autoimmune diseases. Finally, Sjogren's syndrome itself mimics many other disorders, and the dryness is often trivialized as a reaction to a prescribed medication that contains drying agents.

### I Don't Have a Dry Mouth, But I Have Positive Blood Tests and Lip Biopsy. Can I Still Have Sjogren's Syndrome?

Sjogren's syndrome strikes every patient differently. You do not have to have all the symptoms of Sjogren's syndrome to be diagnosed with the disorder. Some persons manifest the symptoms of dryness, while others do not. Remember, Sjogren's syndrome is not just a set of symptoms. It is a systemic autoimmune disease, the course of which is different in every patient.

### The Severity of My Sjogren's Symptoms Has Forced Me to Leave My Job. Since No One Seems to Know About Sjogren's Syndrome, How Can I Collect the Disability Insurance Provided by My Employer?

You should seek counsel as soon as you suspect that you may have a disability claim. Each disability policy is unique and generally requires a trained professional to interpret the coverage. Find an attorney you trust and work with him or her before you take action.

### Is Cosmetic Surgery Recommended for Patients with Sjogren's Syndrome?

According to the outstanding ocular plastic surgeon Perry Garber, MD, when any eyelid surgery is performed, changes can occur in the eyelids that widen the opening between the lids. This results in a decrease in blinking and an increase in tear evaporation. Anyone undergoing eyelid surgery should be evaluated for evidence of dry eyes.

While a moderate dry eye condition does not rule out eyelid surgery, a conservative surgical approach should be taken to ensure the complete closure of the lids and proper blinking. Some surgeons recommend a two-step approach: surgery first on the upper lids to make sure that the patient can tolerate the procedure, followed by surgery on the lower eyelids.

Patients with severe dry eyes are not candidates for elective cosmetic surgery. If they must undergo surgery for significant functional purposes, such as to correct ptosis (drooping of the upper eyelid), it should be conservative.

## Frequently Asked Questions Regarding New Therapies for Sjogren's Syndrome

At the Sjogren's Syndrome Foundation, we frequently receive questions regarding new drugs and products for the treatment of Sjogren's syndrome. Here are a few of the most frequently asked questions and answers.

### Why Isn't There More Research on Sjogren's Syndrome?

There is considerable research into the causes of autoimmune diseases in general and Sjogren's syndrome in particular. Ongoing research takes place at the various institutes of the National Institutes of Health, as well as at some of the finest medical centers in the country.

### Is There a Difference Between Clinical Trials and Research on Sjogren's Syndrome?

The definition of research is much broader than the definition of clinical trials. Basic research involves pure science, innovation, and a search for the truth regarding disease and human biology. At its best, research seeks the truth and is a long, winding path. Clinical trials can be seen as the last steps in the research path and the first steps in the marketing process.

Clinical trials are required by governmental agencies, notably the Food and Drug Administration (FDA), for proof of the efficacy, safety, and correct labeling of any product with pharmaceutical use. These are the last steps a pharmaceutical company must take before a drug or product is marketed by the company and prescribed by a physician.

### Are There Risks Involved in Participating in a Clinical Trial?

Absolutely. A clinical trial is required by the FDA to find out what bad or ineffective outcomes are associated with a new product. These are risks to the patient, and a participant must weigh these before enrollment.

Generally, before starting the trial, a participant signs a release form stating that he or she understands all the risks and is willing to take them. This important document is designed to protect the patient and the pharmaceutical company.

## How Much Do Clinical Trials Cost a Pharmaceutical Company?

Even the most limited trial, such as one seeking only additional labeling, costs pharmaceutical companies millions of dollars. These implementation costs include patient recruitment, physician fees, coordinator fees, indirect costs to institutions, travel, statistical analysis, professional monitoring, legal fees, and so on. The list is staggering from any perspective. These development costs are ultimately borne by consumers once a drug is approved and marketed.

## Who Gains from Clinical Trials?

The goal of the pharmaceutical company is to earn profits from the sale of a medication once it has been approved and marketed. Of course, many patients suffering from a disorder will enjoy relief from their disease. A relatively new and profitable industry, managing clinical trials and analyzing their results, has evolved. A doctor's institution gains too. A practice may expand and gain exposure to new patients. Patients' participation costs (medication cost, administrative costs of medical personnel, etc.) are usually paid by the pharmaceutical company.

## Don't Patients Who Get into a Trial Often Receive Free Medicine and Treatment for Participating?

For a certain percentage of patients, the answer is "yes." Patients interested in enrolling in a trial must remember that only a certain percentage of participants receive the product being tested, and they will not know whether they have received the drug until the study is complete. This may take months and frequently longer. The final phase of a clinical trial requires that some patients receive a placebo (no drug at all) and the others receive the drug being tested. This is called a double-blind study, since neither the participating doctor nor the patient knows what the patient has received until the study has been completed and the code "broken."

## But Why Participate in a Trial If You May Not Get the Drug or Product Being Tested?

A patient who is considering enrolling in a trial must remember that risks should be taken for the benefit of others with the disorder, not just to receive a new therapy. Participating in a clinical trial is an act of compassion for fellow patients. Anyone participating in a clinical study for Sjogren's syndrome should be saluted.

# GLOSSARY

**achlorhydria:** Gastric acid deficiency.

**acne rosacea:** Skin condition characterized by red nose and redness on other parts of the body.

**adenopathy:** A swelling of the lymph nodes. In Sjogren's syndrome, this usually occurs in the neck and jaw region.

**alopecia:** Hair loss.

**alveoli:** Air sacs of the lungs.

**amylase:** An enzyme present in saliva; another form of amylase is produced by the pancreas.

**angular cheilitis:** Sores at the corners of the mouth (angles of the lips).

**antibody:** Substance in the blood that is normally made in response to infection. Also referred to as immunoglobulins such as IgG, IgM, etc.

**antifungal:** Antagonistic (resisting) to fungi.

**antigen(s):** A chemical substance that provokes the production of antibody. In tetanus vaccination, for example, tetanus is the antigen injected to produce antibodies and hence protective immunity to tetanus.

**antimalarial drugs:** Quinine-derived drugs, which were first developed to treat malaria.

**antinuclear antibodies (ANA):** Autoantibodies directed against components in the nucleus of the cell. Screening test for lupus and other connective tissue diseases including Sjogren's syndrome.

**antispasmodic drugs:** Medications that quiet spasms. Usually used in reference to the gastrointestinal tract.

**arteriole:** A very small artery.

**ascites:** An abnormal fluid that collects in the abdomen due to certain liver and other disorders.

**atrophy:** A thinning of the surface; a form of wasting.

**autoantibody:** Antibody that attacks the body's own tissues and organs as if they were foreign.

**autoimmunity:** A state in which the body inappropriately produces antibody against its own tissues. The antigens are components of the body.

**basal (resting) rate:** Unstimulated (used in reference to both tears and salivary flow).

**bolus:** A morsel of food, already chewed, ready to be swallowed.

**bronchi:** Branches of the trachea.

**buffer:** A mixture of acid or base that, when added to a solution, enables the solution to resist changes in the pH that would otherwise occur when acid or alkali is added to it.

**CAH** (chronic active hepatitis): A disorder that occurs when viral hepatitis proceeds in an active state beyond its usual cause.

**calcification:** A process in which tissue or noncellular material in the body becomes hardened as the result of deposits of insoluble calcium salts.

**candidiasis:** Moniliasis. A condition due to an overgrowth of the yeast (fungus) *Candida*.

**cariostatic:** Having the ability to help prevent dental caries.

**celiac disease:** Gluten intolerance.

**CHB** (congenital heart block): A dysfunction of the rate/rhythm conduction system in the fetal or infant heart.

**CNS:** The central nervous system (consisting of the brain and spinal cord).

**connective tissue disease:** A disorder marked by inflammation of the connective tissue (joints, skin, muscles) in multiple areas. In most instances, connective tissue diseases are associated with autoimmunity. Fifty percent of Sjogren's syndrome patients have connective tissue disorders.

**cornea:** The clear "watch crystal" structure covering the pupil and iris (colored portion of the eye). It is composed of several vital layers, all of which are functionally important. The surface layer, or epithelium, is covered by the tears, which lubricate and protect the surface.

**corticosteroid** (steroid, cortisone): A hormone produced by the adrenal cortex gland. Natural adrenal gland hormones have powerful anti-inflammatory activity and are often used in the treatment of severe inflammation affecting vital organs. The many side effects of corticosteroids should markedly curtail their use in mild disorders.

**cryoglobulins:** Protein complexes circulating in the blood that are precipitated during cold.

**cryptogenic cirrhosis (CC):** Liver disease of unknown etiology (origin) in patients with no history of alcoholism or previous acute hepatitis.

**diuretics:** Medications that increase the body's ability to rid itself of fluids.

**double-blind study:** One in which neither the physician nor the patients being treated know whether patients are receiving the active ingredient being tested or a placebo (an inactive substance).

**dysorexia:** Impaired or deranged appetite.

**dysphagia:** Difficulty in swallowing. In Sjogren's syndrome this may be attributable to several causes, among them decreased saliva, infiltration of the glands at the esophageal mucosa, or esophageal webbing.

**dyspnea:** Air hunger resulting in labored or difficult breathing, sometimes accompanied by pain.

**ecchymosis:** A purplish patch caused by oozing of blood into the skin; ecchymoses differ from petechiae in size.

**edema:** Swelling caused by retention of fluid.

**ELISA** (enzyme-linked immunosorbent assay): A very sensitive blood test for detecting the presence of autoantibodies.

**epistaxis:** Nosebleed or hemorrhaging from the nose, which may be caused by dryness of the nasal mucous membrane in Sjogren's syndrome.

**erythema:** A medical term for a red color, usually associated with increased blood flow to an inflamed area, often the skin.

**erythrocyte:** Red blood cell.

**esophagus:** A canal (narrow tube) with muscular walls allowing passage of food from the pharynx, or end of the mouth, to the stomach.

**ESR** (erythrocyte sedimentation rate): Measures the speed at which a column of blood settles. Most common and simple test for inflammation.

**etiology:** The cause(s) of a disease.

**eustachian tube:** The tube running from the back of the nose to the middle ear.

**exocrine glands:** Glands that secrete mucus.

**exocrinopathy:** Disease related to the exocrine glands.

**fibrosis:** Abnormal formation of fibrous tissue.

**fissure:** A crack in the tissue surface (skin, tongue, etc.).

**fluorescein stain:** A dye that stains areas of the eye surface in which cells have been lost.

**gastritis:** Stomach inflammation.

**genetic factors:** Traits inherited from parents, grandparents, and so on.

**gingiva:** The gums.

**gingivitis:** Inflammation of the gums.

**granuloma:** A nodular, inflammatory lesion.

**HLA** (human Leukocyle antigens): A group of genes that governs the ability of lymphocytes, such as T cells and B cells, to respond to foreign and self substances.

**idiopathic:** Of unknown cause.

**immunogenetics:** The study of genetic factors that control the immune response.

**immunoglobulin E:** An antibody associated with allergies.

**immunoglobulins** (gamma globulins): The protein fraction of serum responsible for antibody activity. Measurement of serum immunoglobulin levels can serve as a guide to disease activity in some patients with Sjogren's syndrome.

**immunomodulators:** Medications that affect the body's immune system.

**immunosuppressive agents:** A class of drugs that interferes with the function of cells composing the immune system (see *lymphocyte*). Corticosteroids are immunosuppressive agents. Drugs used in the chemotherapy of malignant disease and in the prevention of transplant rejection are generally immuno-suppressive and occasionally are used to treat severe autoimmune disease.

**incisal:** Cutting edge (of a tooth).

**interstitial:** Supporting structure of the substance of an organ or tissues.

**interstitial nephritis:** Inflammation of the connective tissue of the kidney, usually resulting in mild kidney disease characterized by frequent urination. Interstitial nephritis may be associated with Sjogren's syndrome.

**intraoral:** Inside the mouth.

**KCS** (keratoconjunctivitis sicca): A condition, also called dry eye, that most frequently occurs in women in their 40s and 50s. If it is associated with a dry mouth and/or rheumatoid arthritis, the condition is referred to as Sjogren's syndrome.

**lacrimal:** Relating to the tears.

**lacrimal glands:** Two types of glands that produce tears. Smaller accessory glands in the eyelid tissue produce the tears needed from minute to minute. The main lacrimal glands, located just inside the bony tissue surrounding the eye, produce large amounts of tears.

**larynx:** Voice box.

**latent:** Not manifest but potentially discernible.

**lip biopsy:** Incision of approximately 2 cm on the inside surface of the lower lip and excision of some of the minor salivary glands for microscopic examination and analysis.

**lymph:** A fluid collected from the tissues throughout the body, flowing through the lymph nodes and eventually added to the circulating blood.

**lymphocyte:** A type of white blood cell concerned with antibody production and regulation. Collections of lymphocytes are seen in the salivary glands of Sjogren's syndrome patients.

**lymphoma:** A severe proliferation (increase) of abnormal (malignant) lymphocytes, manifested as cancer of the lymph glands. Although exceedingly rare, lymphoma occurring as a complication of severe Sjogren's syndrome has been identified by immunologists.

**matrix:** The section of the tooth enamel that holds calcium and phosphate minerals.

**MCTD** (mixed connective tissue disease): A connective tissue disease that manifests as an overlap of other connective tissue disorders.

**meibomian glands:** Fat-producing glands in the eyelids that produce an essential component of tears.

**mucin:** Thinnest layer of the tear film; layer closest to the cornea.

**mucolytic agents:** Medications that tend to dissolve mucus. Most patients with dry eyes complain of excess mucous discharge. Some patients may benefit from these medications if other tear film–enhancing drops are not very effective.

**necrosis:** Tissue death.

**nephritis:** An inflammation of the kidneys.

**nonspecific:** Caused by other diseases or multiple factors.

**nonsteroidal anti-inflammatory drugs** (NSAIDS): Chemical derivatives of acetyl-salicylic acid (aspirin), which generally cause fewer side effects (e.g., heart-burn), contain no cortisone, and are used to treat joint pains that occur in rheumatoid arthritis and other connective tissue disorders. Examples include ibuprofen (Motrin), indomethacin (Indocin), sulindac (Clinoril), and pirox-icam (Feldene).

**olfactory:** Relating to the sense of smell.

**ophthalmologist:** A physician who specializes in diseases and surgery of the eye.

**oral mucosa:** The lining (mucous membrane) of the mouth.

**oral soft tissue:** Tongue, mucous lining of the cheeks, and lips.

**otitis:** Inflammation of the ear, which may be marked by pain, fever, abnor-malities of hearing, deafness, tinnitus (a ringing sensation), and vertigo. In Sjogren's syndrome, blockage at eustachian tubes due to infection can lead to conduction deafness and chronic otitis.

**otolaryngologist:** Physician specializing in ear, nose, and throat disorders.

**palate biopsy:** A punch biopsy near the junction of the hard and soft palates to sample the minor salivary glands in that region.

**palpable:** Perceptible to touch.

**parasympathetic nervous system:** The part of the autonomic nervous system whose functions include constriction of the pupils of the eyes, slowing of the heartbeat, and stimulation of certain digestive glands. These nerves originate in the midbrain, the hindbrain, and the sacral region of the spinal cord; impulses are mediated by acetylcholine.

**parotid gland flow:** An empirical quantitative measure of the amount of saliva produced over a certain period of time. Normal parotid gland flow rate is 1.5 ml/min. In Sjogren's syndrome, the flow rate is approximately 0.5 ml/min, with diminution of the flow rate correlating inversely with the severity of disease.

**parotid glands:** One of the three pairs of major salivary glands. They are located in front of the ear.

**PBC** (primary biliary cirrhosis): An impairment of bile excretion secondary to liver inflammation and scarring.

**perforation:** A hole.

**pericarditis:** Inflammation of the lining of the heart.

**periodontitis:** Inflammation of the tissues surrounding and supporting the teeth.

**peripheral nerves:** Those outside the central nervous system.

**petechia:** A small, pinpoint, nonraised, perfectly round, purplish red spot caused by intradermal or submucosal hemorrhaging.

**pharynx:** Throat.

**placebo:** An inactive substance used as a "dummy" medication.

**plaque:** A thin, sticky film that builds up on the teeth, trapping harmful bacteria.

**plasma:** The fluid portion of the circulating blood.

**pleurisy:** Inflammation of the pleura (membrane surrounding the lungs and lining the walls of the rib cavity).

**PM** (polymyositis): A connective tissue disorder characterized by muscle pain and severe weakness secondary to inflammation in the major voluntary muscles.

**psoralen:** A drug administered topically or orally for the treatment of vitiligo (white skin patches caused by loss of pigment).

**puncta:** Small holes in the eyelids that normally drain tears. Patients with severe dry eye benefit from punctal closure, which allows maximal tear preservation.

**purpura:** A condition characterized by hemorrhage into the skin, appearing as crops of petechiae (very small red spots).

**RA** (rheumatoid arthritis): A form of arthritis characterized by inflammation of the joints, stiffness, swelling, cartilaginous hypertrophy, and pain.

**radioactive isotope:** Radioactive material used in diagnostic tests.

**radionuclide studies:** A technique in which radioactive isotopes, such as radiolabeled human serum albumin, are injected into an organ. A gamma scintillation camera, coupled with a digital computer system and a cathode ray display, reads the radioactive emissions. Areas of perfusion will show marked radiographic emissions; areas of obstruction will show no activity.

**Raynaud's phenomenon:** Painful blanching of the fingertips on exposure to cold. This may be seen alone or in association with a connective tissue disease.

**reflux:** A regurgitation due to the return of gas, fluid, or small amount of food from the stomach.

**renal:** Relating to the kidneys.

**RF** (rheumatoid factor): An autoantibody whose presence in the blood usually indicates autoimmune activity.

**rheumatologist:** A physician skilled in the diagnosis and treatment of rheumatic conditions.

**rose bengal:** A dye that stains abnormal or sick cells on the surface of the eye. This diagnostic dye allows the ophthalmologist to follow the treatment of dry eye.

**salicylates:** Aspirin-like drugs. (See *nonsteroidal anti-inflammatory drugs.*)

**salivary scintigraphy:** Measurement of salivary gland function through injection of radioactive material.

**sarcoidosis** (Boeck's disease): A systemic disease with granulomatous (nodular, inflammatory) lesions involving the lungs and, on occasion, the salivary glands, with resulting fibrosis.

**Schirmer test:** The standard objective test to diagnose dry eye. Small pieces of filter paper are placed between the lower eyelid and eyeball and soak the tears for 5 minutes. The value obtained is a rough estimation of tear production in relative terms. Lower values are consistent with dry eye. It is important to emphasize that no single test can be considered diagnostic unless the condition is severe.

**scleroderma:** A connective tissue disorder characterized by thickening and hardening of the skin. Sometimes internal organs (intestines, kidneys) are affected, causing bowel irregularity and high blood pressure.

**serum:** The fluid portion of the blood (obtained after removal of the fibrin clot and blood cells), distinguished from the plasma in the circulation blood.

**sialochemistry:** Measurement of the constituents in saliva.

**sialography:** X-ray examination of the salivary duct system by use of liquid contrast medium. Radiologically sensitive dye is placed into the duct system, outlining the system clearly.

**signs:** Changes that can be seen or measured.

**Sjogren's antibodies:** Abnormal antibodies found in the sera of Sjogren's syndrome patients. These antibodies react with the extracts of certain cells, and a test based on this principle can be helpful in the diagnosis of Sjogren's syndrome. See also SS-A and SS-B.

**Sjogren's syndrome:** A symptom complex of dry eyes, dry mouth, and dryness of other mucous membranes associated with inflammation of the lacrimal and/or salivary glands. It can occur alone (50 percent) or in association with a connective tissue disease.

**SLE** (systemic lupus erythematosus): An inflammatory connective tissue disease.

**SS-A:** Sjogren's syndrome–associated antigen A (anti-Ro).

**SS-B:** Sjogren's syndrome–associated antigen B (anti-La).

**steatorrhea:** Greasy stools (passage of large amounts of fat in the feces, as occurs in pancreatic disease and the malabsorption syndromes).

**steroids:** Cortisone-derived medications.

**sublingual glands:** One of the three pairs of major salivary glands. They are located in the floor of the mouth under the tongue.

**submandibular glands:** One of the three pairs of major salivary glands. They are located below the lower jaw.

**symptoms:** Changes patients feel.

**systemic:** Any process that involves multiple organ systems throughout the body.

**thrush:** A form of candidiasis. Infection of the oral tissues with *Candida albicans*.

**thyroiditis:** A disease in which autoantibodies cause immune system cells (lymphocytes) to destroy the thyroid gland.

**titer:** Test showing the strength or concentration of a particular volume of a solution. Usually refers to amounts of antibody present.

**TMJ** (temporomandibular joint): The joint of the lower jaw where the "ball-and-socket" arrangement is formed by the condyle of the lower jaw (the ball) and the fossa of the temporal bone (the socket). The joint space is filled with synovial or lubricating fluid. This joint and the surrounding synovial tissues may become inflamed if rheumatoid arthritis accompanies Sjogren's syndrome and involves the joint.

**trachea:** Windpipe.

**tracheobronchial tree:** The windpipe and the bronchi into which it subdivides.

**urticaria:** Hives.

**vasculitis:** Inflammation of a blood vessel.

**venule:** A very small vein.

**viscera:** The organs of the digestive, respiratory, urogenital, and endocrine systems, as well as the spleen, heart, and great vessels (blood and lymph ducts).

**vitiligo:** White patches on the skin due to loss of pigment.

**xerophthalmia:** Dry eyes.

**xerostomia:** Dryness of the mouth caused by the arresting of normal salivary secretions. It occurs in diabetes, drug therapy, radiation therapy, and Sjogren's syndrome.

**xylitol:** A sweetening agent with cariostatic properties.

# REFERENCES

## Chapter 9
Flescher E, Talal N: Do viruses contribute to the development of Sjogren's syndrome? Am J Med 90(3):283–285, 1991.

Gudbjornsson B, Bromem JE, Hetta J, Hallgren R: Sleep disturbances in patients with primary Sjogren's syndrome. Br J Rheumatol 32(12):1072–1076, 1993.

Itescu S, Winchester R: Diffuse infiltrating lymphocytosis syndrome: A disorder occurring in human immunodeficiency virus-1 infection that may present as a sicca syndrome. Rheum Dis Clin North Am 18(3):683–697, 1992.

## Chapter 11
Kassan S, Moutsopoulos HM: Sjogren's syndrome, in Paget SA, Field TR (eds): Rheumatic Disorders. Boston, Andover, 1992, pp 185–199.

Kassan S, Talal N: Renal disease with Sjogren's syndrome, in Sjogren's syndrome, Clinical and Immunological Aspects, Talal N, Moutsopoulos HM, and Kassan S, Sjogren's syndrome (eds), Berlin, Springer-Verlag, 1987, pp 96–101.

## Chapter 16
Bengtsson A, Backman E, Lindblom B, Skogh T: Long-term follow-up of fibromyalgia patients: Clinical symptoms, muscular function, laboratory tests—an eight-year comparison study. Musculoskeletal Pain 2:67–80, 1994.

Bennett RM: A multidisciplinary approach to treating fibromyalgia, in Vaeroy M, Merskey M (eds): Progress in Fibromyalgia and Myofascial Pain. Amsterdam, New York, London, Tokyo, Elsevier, 1993, p 393.

Bennett RM, Clark SR, Campbell SM, Ingram SB, Burckhardt CS, Nebon DL, Porter JM: Symptoms of Raynaud's syndrome in patients with fibromyalgia. A study utilizing the Nielsen test, digital photoplethysmography, and measurements of platelet alpha 2-adrenergic receptors. Arthritis Rheum 34:264–269, 1991.

Bennett RM, Gatter RA, Campbell SM, Andrews RP, Clark SR, Scarola JA: A comparison of cyclobenzaprine and placebo in the management of fibrositis. A double-blind controlled study. Arthritis Rheum 31:1535–1542, 1988.

Blasberg B, Chalmers A: Temporomandibular pain and dysfunction syndrome associated with generalized musculoskeletal pain: A retrospective study. J Rheumatol Suppl 19:87–90, 1989.

Bonafedo RP, Downey DC, Bennett RM: An association of fibromyalgia with primary Sjogren's syndrome: A prospective study of 72 patients. J Rheumatol 22:133–136, 1995.

Branco J, Atalaia A, Paiva T: Sleep cycles and alpha-delta sleep in fibromyalgia syndrome. J Rheumatol 21:1113–1117, 1994.

Burckhardt CS, Clark SR, Bennett RM: Fibromyalgia and quality of life: A comparative analysis. J Rheumatol 20:475–479, 1993.

Burckhardt CS, O'Reilly CA, Wiens AN, Clark SR, Campbell SM, Bennett RM: Assessing depression in fibromyalgia patients. Arthritis Care Res 7:35–39, 1994.

Caidahl K, Lurie M, Bake B, Johansson G, Wetterquist H: Dyspnoea in chronic primary fibromyalgia. Ann Intern Med 226:265–270, 1989.

Carette S, Bell MJ, Reynolds WJ, Harsoui B, McCain GA, Bykerk VP, Edworthy SM, Baron M, Koehler BE, Fam AG, Bellamy N, Guimont C: Comparison of amitriptyline, cyclobenzaprine, and placebo in the treatment of fibromyalgia. Arthritis Rheum 37:32–40, 1994.

Clark S, Tindall E, Bennett RM: A double blind crossover trial of prednisone versus placebo in the treatment of fibrositis. J Rheumatol 12:980–983, 1985.

Clark SR: Prescribing exercise for fibromyalgia patients. Arthritis Care Res 7:221–225, 1994.

Deodhar AA, Fisher RA, Blacker CVR, Woolf AD: Fluid retention syndrome and fibromyalgia. Bri Rheumatol 33:576–582, 1994.

Dinerrnan H, Goldenberg DL, Felson DT: A prospective evaluation of 118 patients with the fibromyalgia syndrome: Prevalence of Raynaud's phenomenon, sicca symptoms, ANA, low complement, and Ig deposition at the dermalepidermal junction. J Rheumatol 13:368–373, 1986.

Felson DT, Goldenberg DR: The natural history of fibromyalgia. Arthritis Rheum 29:1522–1526, 1986.

Gerster JC, Hadj Djilani A: Hearing and vestibular abnormalities in primary fibrositis syndrome. J Rheumatol 11:678–680, 1984.

Goldenberg DL: A review of the role of tricyclic medications in the treatment of fibromyalgia syndrome. J Rheumatol Suppl 19:137–139, 1989.

Gowera WR: Lumbago: Its lessons and analogies. BMJ 1:117–121, 1904.

Henriksson C, Gundmark I, Bengtsson A, Ek AC: Living with fibromyalgia. Consequences for everyday life. Clin J Pain 8:138–144, 1992.

Ledingham I, Doberty S, Doberty M: Primary fibromyalgia syndrome—an outcome study. Br J Rheumatol 32:139–142, 1993.

Middleton GD, McFarlin JE, Lipsky PE: The prevalence and clinical impact of fibromyalgia in systemic lupus erythematosus. Arthritis Rheum 37:1181–1188, 1994.

Pellegrino MJ: Atypical chest pain as an initial presentation of primary fibromyalgia. Arch Phys Med Rehabil 71:526–528, 1990.

Reilly PA, Littlejohn GO: Peripheral arthralgic presentation of fibrositis/fibromyalgia syndrome. J Rheumatol 19:281–283, 1992.

Russell U, Fletcher EM, Michalek JE, McBroom PC, Hester GG: Treatment of primary fibrositis/fibromyalgia syndrome with ibuprofen and alprazolam: A double-blind, placebo-controlled study. Arthritis Rheum 34:552–560, 1991.

Schned ES, Williams DN: Special concerns in Lyme disease. Seropositivity with vague symptoms and development of fibrositis. Postgrad Med 91:65–68, 70, 1992.

Simms RW, Ferrante N, Craven DE: High prevalence of fibromyalgia syndrome (FMS) in human immunodeficiency virus type I (HIV) infected patients with polyarthralgia. Arthritis Rheum 33:S136, 1990.

Travell JG, Simons DG: Myofacial Pain and Dysfunction: The Trigger Point Manual. Baltimore, Williams & Wilkins, 1983.

Veal D, Kavanagh G, Fielding JF, Fitzgerald O: Primary fibromyalgia and the irritable bowel syndrome: Different expressions of a common pathogenetic process. Br J Rheumatol 30:220–222, 1991.

Vitali C, Tavoni A, Neri R, Castrogiovanni P, Pasero G, Bombardieri S: Fibromyalgia features in patients with primary Sjogren's syndrome. Evidence of a relationship with psychological depression. Scand J Rheumatol 18:21–27, 1989.

Wallace DJ: Genitourinary manifestations of fibrositis: An increased association with the female urethral syndrome. J Rheumatol 17:238–239, 1990.

Waylonis GW, Ronan PG, Gordon C: A profile of fibromyalgia in occupational environments. Am J Phys Med Rehabil 73:112–115, 1994.

Wolfe F, Cathey MA, Kleinheksel SM: Fibrositis (fibromyalgia) in rheumatoid arthritis. J Rheumatol 11:814–818, 1984.

Wolfe F, Ross K, Anderson J, Russell IJ, Hebert L: The prevalence and characteristics of fibromyalgia in the general population. Arthritis Rheum 38:19–28, 1995.

Wolfe F, Smythe HA, Yunua MB, Bennett RM, Bombardier C, Goldeoberg DL, Tugwell P, Campbell SM, Abeleo M, Clarlc P, Fam AG, Farber SJ, Fiechtner JJ, Franiclin CM, Gatter RA, Hamaty D, Lessud I, Lichtbmun AS, Masi AT, McCain GA, Reynolds WJ, Romano TJ, Russell LJ, Sheon RP: The American College of Rheumatology 1990 criteria for the classification of fibromyalgia: Report of the Multicenter Criteria Committee. Arthritis Rheum 33:160–172, 1990.

Yunus M, Masi AT, Calabro JJ, Miller KA, Feigenbaum SL: Primary fibromyalgia (fibrositis): Clinical study of 50 patients with matched normal controls. Semin Arthritis Rheum 1:151–171, 1981.

### Chapter 18

Buyon JP: Neonatal lupus syndromes, in Lahita R (ed): Systemic Lupus Erythematousus. New York, Churchill Livingstone, 1992.

Buyon JP, Winchester RJ, Slade SG, Arnett F, Copel J, Friedman D, Lockshin MD: Identification of mothers at risk for congenital heart block and other neonatal lupus syndromes in their children: Comparison of ELISA and immunoblot to measure Anti-SSA/Ro and Anti-SSB/La antibodies. Arthritis Rheum 36:1263–1273, 1993.

Lee LA: Neonatal lupus erythematosus. J Invest Dermatol 100:9s–13s, 1993.

Rider L, Buyon J, Rutledge J, Sherry D: Postnatal treatment of neonatal lupus: Case report and review of the literature. J Rheumatol 20:1208–1211, 1993.

Silverman ED: Congenital heart block and neonatal lupus erythematosus: Prevention is the goal. J Rheumatol 20:1101–1104, 1993.

Waltuck J, Buyon JP: Autoantibody-associated congenital heart block: Outcome in mothers and children. Ann Intern Med 120:544–555, 1994.

### Chapter 22
Brodnitz FS: Keep Your Voice Healthy. Boston, College-Hill Press, Little, Brown, 1988.

Cooper M: Change Your Voice, Change Your Life. New York, Harper & Row, 1985.

### Chapter 24
Cros DA, Krupkin T: Implications of the effect of general anesthesia on basal tear production. Anesth Analg 56:35–38, 1977.

Fukui A, Makashima Y, Kimura K: Anesthetic management of a patient with Sjogren's syndrome. MASUI 40(4):627–631, 1991.

Murrin KR: Causes of difficult intubation, in Lalto IP, Rosen M (eds): Difficulties in Tracheal Intubation. Philadelphia, WB Saunders, 1985, pp 85–86.

Phillips S, Hutchinson S, Davidson T: Preoperative drinking does not affect gastric contents. Br J Anaesth 70:6–9, 1993.

Takahashi S, Ogasawara H, Tsubo T, et al: Anesthetic management of a patient with Sjogren's syndrome and pulmonary fibrosis. MASUI 39(10):1393–1396, 1990.

# INDEX

**A**

acetylcholine, 203

acetylsalicylic acid. *See* aspirin

achalasia, in Sjogren's syndrome, 88, 94, 95

achlorhydria, definition of, 199

acidosis, in kidney disease, 99, 100

acinar cells, 19

acne rosacea, definition of, 199

acquired immunodeficiency syndrome. *See* AIDS

acupuncture, for fibromyalgia, 123

adenopathy, definition of, 199

adrenal glands, cortisol production by, 149, 151, 200

Advil. *See* ibuprofen

Aerobid, for tracheobronchitis, 89

African Americans, Sjogren's syndrome in, 20, 26

age, Sjogren's syndrome and, 24

aging, hearing loss in, 65

AIDS
    salivary protection against, 56
    Sjogren's syndrome and, 193

air conditioning, effects on eyes, 49

air currents, effects on eyes, 49

air travel
    comfort tips for, 68, 188, 191–192
    dryness from, 67

albumin, in urine, 100

alcohol, 30
    avoidance in corticosteroid therapy, 152
    dryness from, 185
    in methotrexate therapy, 154
    pancreatitis from, 96
    voice problems from, 165

alendronate, for osteoporosis, 152

allergies
    allergen avoidance in, 114–115

causes of, 114

dryness from, 31, 33, 67

to oil-based vaginal lubricants, 130

Sjogren's syndrome and, 113–117

symptoms of, 114

tests for, 114

treatments for, 116–117

alopecia. *See* hair loss

alpha channel blockers, for Raynaud's phenomenon, 77

alprazolam, for fibromyalgia sleep disorder, 122

altruistic cell death. *See* apoptosis

alveoli
    definition of, 199
    in interstitial pneumonia, 90

Alzheimer's disease, estrogen replacement therapy and, 131

American College of Rheumatology, 118

aminophylline, for tracheobronchitis, 89

amitriptyline, for fibromyalgia, 121

amoxicillin, allergic reaction to, 170

ampicillin, allergic reaction to, 170

amylase
    pancreatic production of, 54, 96, 199
    in saliva, 54, 96, 199

amyloidosis
    eye and mouth dryness in, 5
    saliva decrease in, 60
    in Sjogren's syndrome, 87

ANA. *See* antinuclear antibodies (ANA)

anaerobic pneumonia, causes and treatment of, 87–88

anagen, of normal hair, 111

Anaprox. *See* naproxen sodium

androgens. *See* male hormones

anemia
    in rheumatoid arthritis, 72
    in Sjogren's syndrome with vasculitis, 81